The Unbalanced Mind

MAPS OF THE MIND
Steven Rose, General Editor

MAPS OF THE MIND
Steven Rose, General Editor

Pain: The Science of Suffering
Patrick Wall

The Making of Intelligence
Ken Richardson

How Brains Make Up Their Minds
Walter J. Freeman

Sexing the Brain
Lesley Rogers

Intoxicating Minds: How Drugs Work
Ciaran Regan

How to Build a Mind: Toward Machines with Imagination
Igor Aleksander

The Aging Brain
Lawrence Whalley

The Unbalanced
Mind

Julian Leff

Columbia University Press
New York

Columbia University Press
Publishers Since 1893
New York   Chichester, West Sussex

Library of Congress Cataloging-in-Publication Data
Leff, Julian P.
    The unbalanced mind / Julian Leff.
      p. cm. — (Maps of the mind)
    Includes bibliographical references and index.
    ISBN 0–231–12026–5 (cloth : alk. paper)
      1. Mental illness.   2. Mental illness—Etiology. 3. Mental illness—
    Treatment. 4. Mental illness—Social aspects.   I. Title.   II. Series.
    RC454 .L375 2001
    616.89—dc21
    2001028993

⊗
Casebound editions of Columbia University Press books are printed on
permanent and durable acid-free paper.

Printed in Great Britain

c 10 9 8 7 6 5 4 3 2 1

First published by Weidenfeld & Nicolson Ltd., London

Acknowledgements

I am grateful to my wife, Joan Raphael-Leff, for providing loving companionship during many hours of writing and for acting as a living thesaurus and a constructive critic. Thanks are also due to her mother, Fan Raphael, for researching Shabbetai Zvi, the false Messiah. The following friends and relatives read through various drafts of the book and provided me with invaluable guidance and comments: Michael Dorfman, Cheli Duran, Alex Leff, Jessa Leff, Andrew Szmidla. I am very grateful to Steven Rose for initiating this project and for steering it through to a successful conclusion.

Contents

Introduction

The so-called 'master plan' of the human genome has recently been unfolded in its entirety. Some hail this as the key that will unlock a complete understanding of the human mind and hence of human behaviour. This is a chilling vision, reminiscent of *A Clockwork Orange*, as it implies that substituting for, or transposing, the basic units of the master plan will alter human behaviour to suit the manipulator of the molecules. My purpose in writing this book is to temper this Orwellian view of the future.

I grew up in an environment of optimism that improving the environment, both physical and social, would change human behaviour for the better. My mother was a committed Marxist who believed that the establishment of communism in Russia and China heralded the dawn of Utopia. My father, also a Marxist, worked as a public health doctor, ensuring that drinking water and food were safe, that sewage was properly disposed of, that factories were safe for the workforce, and that there were sufficient day-nursery places for young children. So convinced was he of the eventual effectiveness of these kinds of environmental improvements that he tried to dissuade me from studying medicine, arguing that doctors who treated individuals would soon be redundant. The year 1956 was a disaster for the utopian vision of my parents, with Khrushchev's revelations of Stalin's enormities and the Soviet invasion of Hungary. Their activities for the

Party virtually ceased, although my father's deep commitment to the National Health Service, which he helped to establish, remained undiminished.

I had never shared my parents' illusions about Soviet communism, being turned off by any autocratic system, but their beliefs about the overriding importance of the social environment were in my bones – not my genes, since my grandfather, who lived with us throughout my childhood, was a staunch capitalist! It was not surprising, then, that when I qualified as a psychiatrist and was looking around for a job, I jumped at the offer of a position in the social psychiatry unit at the Institute of Psychiatry in London. Not only was I attracted by the intellectual challenge of a research career, but the focus of the unit and its director, John Wing, appeared entirely consonant with my own views of society. I was understandably surprised, therefore, when the first study John Wing directed me to design and conduct was a test of the value of medication to prevent repeated attacks of schizophrenia. It had already been proved that chlorpromazine (Largactil) and trifluoperazine (Stelazine) helped patients with delusions and hallucinations to recover from their illness, but it was unknown whether it was useful for them to continue to take these medicines once they were well. I tackled the problems of designing a trial of preventive medication with a will, but was determined to include some measure of the social environment. Reading the literature, I discovered that social stress in the form of sudden happenings, known as life events, provoked attacks of schizophrenia (more about this later), so I included measures of life events in the study.

My conclusion at the end of the trial was that continuing with medication following recovery did reduce the chance of a further attack of illness.[1] The inclusion of the life events measure added another dimension to our understanding of the results. A similar trial was being conducted by my colleague Steven Hirsch, who was testing the value of preventive medication given by long-acting injection.[2] We were able to pool the data from the two trials to look at the effects of life events in a reasonably large group of patients. We found that eighty-nine per cent of patients whose illness returned while they were taking medication had experienced a life event in the five weeks before the relapse, compared with only twenty-seven per cent of those on drugs who remained well throughout the trial.[3] This showed that unexpected events causing a high level of stress could break through the protective barrier built up by the medication.

My first experience of conducting research in the unit gave me an understanding of the importance of including both a biological and a social perspective on psychiatric problems. In this book I do not challenge the importance of the biological basis of mental activity, but as far as possible show how it can be integrated with our understanding of the impact of the social environment. A substantial amount of research has accumulated over many decades revealing the importance to mental wellbeing of the network of relationships that each of us experiences as centred on ourselves. It appears to radiate outwards from us, encompassing (with increasing distance) family, friends, workmates, shopkeepers and acquaintances. This is, of course, an illusion stemming from our egocentric view of the world. Seen from above, there would be a continuous network with no centre, but with areas of greater and lesser density, constituting an entire culture. In the course of the book I will focus on smaller and larger sections of the network, from the most intimate relationships to the whole culture.

I will also present material on different types of psychiatric conditions. Mental illness takes many forms ranging from emotional distress, affecting most of us at some time in our life, to psychotic illnesses such as manic-depression and schizophrenia, which appear in about one per cent of the population. It is important to appreciate a general distinction between neuroses and psychoses. Neuroses represent an intensification of emotions that all humans feel, such as depression and anxiety, to the point when they interfere with daily life. People with psychoses can also have high levels of depression and anxiety, but in addition they have experiences that are out of the ordinary, such as developing beliefs that are not shared by their own social group (delusions), or hearing voices and seeing visions that others do not hear or see (hallucinations). The main psychoses are schizophrenia and manic-depressive illness. Depression is awkward because it runs across the boundaries between neuroses and psychoses and hence has always faced psychiatrists with the challenge of knowing how to fit it into their systems of classification. The social, political and economic forces that influence psychiatrists' choice of pigeonholes will be explored later.

Both psychoses and neuroses feature several times in the story as they serve to advance my argument about the importance of the social environment for the whole range of psychiatric conditions. The sequence of the narrative is driven more by my exploration of different features of the social environment than by any particular classification of illnesses. Hence I will sometimes use schizophrenia to illustrate a point, and sometimes depression or another neurosis. When I began my research career in 1968 there were six research units supported by the Medical Research Council or the Department of Health, dedicated to investigating social issues in psychiatry. Today there is none. Biological research is generally seen to be the best bet for finding the answers to people's mental problems, and since the technical equipment and support needed are very expensive, there are few funds left over for social research. By the end of the book, I hope you will have gained an appreciation of the need for a balance between biological and social explanations for the vagaries of the human mind.

Chapter 1

How Blue is Blue?

We all have times when we feel miserable, often for no apparent reason. We talk of feeling 'blue', of being 'down in the dumps', or 'under the weather'. We proffer explanations which have no plausibility, such as 'I got out of bed the wrong side this morning'. Sometimes a low mood is an obvious consequence of a major disruption in our life, such as the break-up of a relationship or the death of someone we love. Our friends and relatives would be concerned for us if we became sad following such an event, but would not think of us as ill.

Andrew held a responsible job in a wines and spirits firm in which he had worked for twenty years. He had another fifteen years before retirement and enjoyed his work. The firm was taken over by a large corporation and he was declared redundant without notice. He was shocked and could not believe it had happened to him. He lay awake at night experiencing a mixture of misery and rage. He went off his food and moped around all day doing nothing. His wife and friends rallied round and encouraged him to think of alternative jobs. After a few weeks of being paralysed by his situation, he began to look for a position and realised that there were a number of options open to him.

How intense does our misery have to become before a doctor would consider it to be an illness and diagnose depression?

Should Andrew have been treated with antidepressants? The problem facing the doctor is that there is no test that will reveal whether the person is suffering from a depressive illness. In fact this problem affects the whole of psychiatry. There are no distinctive abnormalities of the blood, the body chemistry, the electrical activity of the brain or its appearance that can serve to diagnose any of the common psychiatric disorders. Numerous studies have identified changes in the structure of the brain and in the form of the brain waves in people with schizophrenia, while depressed people have been found to have abnormalities in the amounts of certain chemical transmitters in the brain. However, many people with these illnesses do not differ from healthy people in their brain structure and function, while some people with no psychiatric symptoms show the same abnormalities as the patients. This large overlap between healthy and ill people makes it impossible for the psychiatrist to use these brain changes to make a diagnosis.

Exciting new methods continue to be developed to visualise the structure and function of the brain. Although beautiful pictures are produced by these techniques, they have not advanced to the stage where they can be used to back up a diagnosis. There is a widespread belief among psychiatrists and researchers that this goal is not far off, but no one can be sure that it will ever be achieved.

Serendipity and psychiatric treatments

We can ask how far depression might be explained by changes in the functioning of the brain. Our thoughts, feelings and actions are obviously the result of brain activity at one level; but it does not follow that depression can be explained by changes in the way the brain works, or that reversing these changes would necessarily cure the depression. Antidepressant drugs were introduced in the 1950s and have become one of the most widely prescribed class of psychiatric treatments. But they were not designer drugs, chemically crafted to correct a known abnormality in the brain. Far from it: one of the first groups of antidepressants was developed from isoniazid, an antibiotic used for tuberculosis, because it was noticed that patients treated with this medication appeared to gain relief from the depressing effects of their chronic ill-health. Many of the treatments introduced into psychiatry have their origins in serendipity, including another frequently prescribed group of drugs, the tricyclic anti-depressants. The first representative of this group, imi-pramine (UK trade name Tofranil), was synthesised in the 1940s as one of a series of antihistamines, sedatives and painkillers. It was recommended as a treatment to calm agitated psychotic patients, but in 1958 it was found to do little for these patients, but to have effects in relieving depression.

How the brain sends messages

A recent development in the drug treatment of depression is the introduction of a family of drugs called specific serotonin reuptake inhibitors (SSRIs). Signals are sent between brain cells (neurons) by chemicals known as transmitters. One of the most common chemical messengers in the brain is serotonin, the chemical name of which is 5-hydroxy-tryptamine. Serotonin is also found in the gut, and in bananas as well! One theory is that depression is caused by an inherited lack of serotonin in the brain.

The brain is an efficient organ and does not waste chemicals. When a transmitter has been released and has activated a receptor on the adjacent brain cell, any excess is transferred back into the nerve ending ('reuptake'), to be recirculated later. There is a specific serotonin reuptake process which works through a transporter molecule. The use of an SSRI to prevent this molecule transporting the excess serotonin back into the nerve ending results in an increase in the amount of serotonin washing around the neurons. Since serotonin activates a particular class of brain cells, this increase is believed to counteract the sluggishness of these neurons in depression. The drug fluoxetine, better known as Prozac, is an SSRI, but is only one of a whole family of antidepressants with similar effects on the level of serotonin in the brain. Although these drugs specifically block the reuptake of serotonin, they are not like so-called 'smart' bombs which pinpoint targets, since they affect the chemical process wherever it occurs in the body. As there are many serotonin receptors in the gut, 'collateral damage' occurs in the form of unpleasant intestinal side-effects, such as nausea and diarrhoea.

Maternity blues

One of the pieces of evidence put forward for a biochemical origin for depression is the occurrence of 'maternity blues' in the mother immediately after the birth of a baby. Dramatic hormonal changes occur in the mother's body with the expulsion of the placenta and the onset of lactation. The mother's mood swings up and down for the first few days after the birth and bouts of tearfulness are common, the lowest point being between the third and fifth postnatal day. There is, however, a great deal of individual variation: some mothers do not experience a low mood, and most of those who do level out in a few days, while a small group go on to develop a full-blown depressive illness. The proportions at each stage have been determined by a group of researchers working in a maternity hospital in Paris in 1997.[4] They gave two questionnaires to 126 women who gave birth at their hospital. The first questionnaire was designed to detect maternity blues and was filled in by the mothers on the third or fourth day after delivery. The second was aimed at picking up depression of clinical severity and was completed eight months after the birth. The mothers were asked to respond to the questions according to their feelings in the previous eight days. Almost exactly half the women reported experiencing maternity blues: of those with moderate blues, sixteen per cent were diagnosed as depressed eight months later, whereas of those with severe blues, the proportion who became depressed reached twenty-eight per cent. Of the sixty-four women who escaped the blues, only one was rated as depressed at eight months. These figures establish a strong link between maternity blues and later depression, and suggest that there may be a common biochemical basis for the two conditions, but that is not the whole story.

In order to discover why some women were more likely than others to develop depression after a birth, in the 1980s Channi Kumar and Kay Robson in London investigated a number of factors that might be responsible.[5] One of their findings was unexpected: women who had had an induced abortion were more prone to postnatal depression than those without this history. This was true even if the abortion had been many years earlier. It is inconceivable that the hormonal changes following an abortion could linger for years, so that the most plausible explanation is that the psychological impact of the abortion was reactivated by the birth of a baby, intensifying the biochemical changes occurring at that time. This is not the only environmental factor to be implicated in the origin of postnatal depression. Other researchers have stressed the importance of difficult living conditions, socio-economic problems, and lack of emotional support from the child's father and the wider social network. These aspects of environmental stress have also been shown to contribute to the causation of depression unrelated to childbirth.

Genes and the mind

Research on the impact of the social environment on a person's feelings, thoughts and behaviour has been overshadowed in recent years by the conviction held by many brain scientists that all mental activity will sooner or later be explicable in terms of genes and molecules. It is undeniable that the infant science of molecular genetics has already led to huge leaps in our understanding of certain physical diseases, such as cystic fibrosis. Identification of the specific sequence of the particular gene that gives rise to the abnormality raises the exciting possibility of correcting the problem at source through genetic engineering. There have been extravagant claims to have found a gene for homosexuality and for child abuse, but these have not been replicated by other scientists. A number of different genes have been linked with schizophrenia, for which the evidence for an inherited basis is strong. However, no single gene has been identified as the prime cause of the illness and some research groups have failed to find the same links as others. It seems likely that a number of different genes acting in concert are risk factors for the brain problems underlying schizophrenia. The inheritance of height, for example, is known to depend on the interaction of a number of genes. We have to conclude that, so far, the bright promise of molecular genetics has failed to illuminate any psychiatric condition beyond identifying some genes as potential risk factors.

Public attitudes

It is intriguing that the scientists' love affair with biological determinism has not influenced the views of the public on the causes and treatment of mental illness. Numerous surveys of public opinion over the years have come up with the same finding: stress is held to be the prime cause of the entire range of psychiatric conditions from anxiety to schizophrenia. This belief has a long pedigree: Shakespeare in *The Comedy of Errors* has an abbess question the wife of a man deemed to be mad as follows: 'Hath he not lost much wealth by wrack of sea? Buried some dear friend? Hath not else his eye stray'd his affection in unlawful love, a sin prevailing much in youthful men, who give their eyes the liberty of gazing? Which of these sorrows is he subject to?' When asked about the treatment of mental illnesses, the public favour social support and talking therapies over physical treatments, and are generally very wary of antidepressants, which they view as addictive. This mistaken conviction may well have been implanted by the widely disseminated information on the addictive nature of the minor tranquillisers, such as chlordiazepoxide (Librium) and diazepam (Valium), which for a time were extensively prescribed to depressed patients by primary care doctors.

The term 'addiction' is used loosely by the public, as in 'addicted to shopping'. In medicine it covers both a psychological reliance on a drug, and also a physical need for it, which develops over time with certain drugs. Thus a person who is physically addicted to alcohol will develop the 'shakes' after a day or so of not drinking, or even start to see small animals crawling over the walls and floor (delirium tremens or 'the DTs'). The minor tranquillisers can produce a physical addiction even at small doses, so that a patient who stops taking them will experience very unpleasant sensations. Antidepressants never produce physical addiction, and most patients can stop them without ill effects, although a few find that their depression returns soon after. An educational campaign mounted recently in Britain by the Royal College of Psychiatrists and the Royal College of General Practitioners, which was partly aimed at lessening public prejudice against antidepressants, made only a small impact. We shall encounter this prejudice and its effects on compliance with drug prescriptions later, in our discussion of treatments for depression.

Measuring depression across cultures

Up to this point we have sidestepped the issue referred to in the title of this chapter, namely how miserable do you have to be before you cross the threshold into the domain of depression that requires treatment. We have to confront this question before discussing the social factors leading to depression, since it is fundamental to any comparison of results across studies. In 1988 I compiled a review of a large number of studies of the frequency of depression in the general population. These surveys had been carried out in many different countries, both developed, such as Britain, Greece and Argentina, and developing, such as Taiwan, India and Uganda. A variety of interview schedules and questionnaires had been used, making direct comparison of results very problematic. Imagine using a ruler marked in inches in one country and one marked in centimetres in another, and then attempting to compare the two sets of measurements without knowing how to convert from inches to centimetres. A more useful approach is to employ the same instrument for measuring depression in both countries, but unless the people speak the same language, it is necessary to translate it. This is not as straightforward as it might seem, since the accuracy of the translation has to be verified. The technique that has been developed for this purpose is called back-translation. One person translates the instrument from language A into language B. A second person, independent of the first, then translates the instrument back from language B to language A. The two versions in language A are then compared for discrepancies, revealing any faulty translations into B, which can then be corrected. Even this careful procedure is not foolproof, since it fails to detect problems with the usage of particular words. An example is provided by Lyn Gillis and his colleagues who translated a psychiatric assessment interview, the Present State Examination, from English into Xhosa, a South African language, in 1982.[6] The Xhosa term for emotion, *inimba*, appeared to be correct when back-translated into English, but when the Xhosa version was used it emerged that the term denoted a feeling state that can only be experienced by women.

Very few of the studies I reviewed had used the same instrument plus the technique of back-translation. The frequency of depression and other neuroses ranged from a low of 0.8 per 1000 people in an aboriginal population on the island of Taiwan to a high of 287 per 1000 for women in Buenos Aires. It is unlikely that human populations differ so remarkably in their liability to neuroses, so that much of the variation can be attributed to problems of measurement. In support of this interpretation are the findings from a study conducted in 1979 in Uganda by John Orley and John Wing.[7] John Orley has an unusual combination of training in both anthropology and psychiatry. He lived in a village in Uganda for eighteen months and learned the local language, Buganda. He then translated the Present State Examination interview into Buganda, following which his version was checked by back-translation. He surveyed two villages with this measuring instrument and then compared the rates of neuroses with those derived from a survey in London. The rate for Ugandan women was 269 per 1000 compared with 106 per 1000 for women in London. The rates for men were 174 and 58 per 1000 respectively. While the rates are two and a half to three times higher for Ugandan women and men, this is a credible difference compared with the 300-fold variation between the highest and lowest rates in my survey of the literature.

Measuring symptoms

We can learn a great deal about the measurement of depression by considering the construction of the Present State Examination (PSE). In the absence of laboratory tests, the only information available on which to base a diagnosis is the person's experiences and behaviour. Experience can be tapped only by questioning the person directly, while behaviour can be observed by the interviewer, supplemented by accounts given by people who know the person well (usually relatives). The techniques of exploring the person's experiences and classifying them derive from the science of phenomenology, and were applied definitively to psychiatry by the German psychiatrist, Karl Jaspers, whose textbook was published in 1913. The PSE provides the interviewer with a skeletal structure of questions which prompt a dialogue with the interviewee. The purpose of the dialogue is to explore and clarify the person's experiences in order to determine whether they fit the categories of symptoms built into the PSE.

Here is an example of a dialogue with a patient generated by the section of the PSE which covers anxiety:

Interviewer: Have there been times lately when you've been very anxious or frightened?
Patient: Yes, there have.
Interviewer: Have you tended to get very anxious in certain special situations, such as travelling, or crossing the road?
Patient: Yes, I find it hard to go out.
Interviewer: Does it bother you to cross open spaces like parks or squares, or do you get anxious in shops or on buses?
Patient: I can walk across a square if there aren't many people around, but I can't stand being in a shop with crowds of people.
Interviewer: Is it the same problem with a crowded bus?
Patient: Oh, yes. If a bus comes along that's full of people, I'll wait for the next one in the hope that it will be less crowded.
Interviewer: Do you find it easier to go out at night?
Patient: Yes, I do all my shopping at late-night supermarkets, because there aren't many other people around and I don't have to stand in a queue with other customers.

The interviewer's detective work establishes that the patient has anxiety that is provoked by being in crowds, which is classified as a phobia. The interview schedule is accompanied by a glossary which defines each symptom precisely and gives examples. People's experiences rarely fit neatly into predetermined categories, so the interviewer often has to judge whether an experience approximates closely enough to a definition to be rated as a symptom. In making this judgement, the interviewer needs to take into account both the intensity of the experience and its frequency. To take the pertinent example of depressed mood, the questions that need to be asked are: how often during the past month has the person felt depressed? Has it occurred every day or only once or twice a week? How long does it last? Does the person cry or feel like crying? Here I should comment that the interviewer must gauge the answer in the light of the person's gender and culture. It is more acceptable for women to cry than men, except on the football field, where the whole range of emotions gains much freer expression than in everyday life. Furthermore, people from northern Europe are less expressive than those from southern Europe.

Other questions that will help the interviewer decide on the degree of depression are: does the low mood fluctuate in intensity or remain at the same level? Can it be relieved by anything, for example, can a friend cheer the person up? Has all enjoyment of life ceased or are there still things that can be enjoyed? How bad is the feeling when it is at its worst? This last question differs in kind from the others as it is not factual, but requires the person to find their own words to describe their experience. Expressions such as 'it feels like a dark cloud', 'I feel paralysed by it', or, paradoxically, 'it is an indescribable feeling', indicate a severity of mood that is well beyond ordinary sadness.

Here are some other descriptions by patients from interviews with the PSE which convey the experience of depression:

'I just can't make myself do anything. My brain isn't working at all. My mind has gone dead. I've just become like this. I can't say to myself, "do this, do that". I'm just not how I used to be.'

'I'm fighting the tiredness and the depression. Trying to organise my life. Everything's been such a muddle. I spent days lying in bed. The tiredness was getting me down. I have been crying incessantly.'

'I get gloomy over anything I read in the newspapers. I dreamed about my father dying. I feel everyone would be better off without me.'

'Sometimes I feel low and I cry quite a lot. I can see no future and I feel completely trapped. There's an emptiness inside me. Nothing means anything. I feel as if I'm sinking.'

The presence of depressed mood is obviously essential for a diagnosis of a depressive illness, but there are other symptoms that often accompany it and that contribute to the diagnosis. These include poor appetite and weight loss, difficulty in sleeping, loss of interest in sex, slowness in thinking and moving about, lack of energy, and poor concentration. The PSE requires the interviewer to enquire about each symptom in some detail to establish its presence, as in the example above. Consequently the interview is long and demanding for both interviewer and subject. Various short cuts have been developed in the form of self-report questionnaires, which do not require the presence of a professional person and can even be sent by post or be filled in on a computer. They cannot achieve the same degree of accuracy as an interview like the PSE, but they are practical alternatives for large-scale surveys. Some attempt to cover a wide range of symptoms of neurosis, such as the General Health Questionnaire developed by David Goldberg in 1970 while he was in Manchester,[8] while others have a narrow focus on symptoms of depression and/or anxiety, such as the Hamilton Rating Scale for Depression and the Beck Depression Inventory. A couple of questions from the latter will convey the style of these questionnaires.

B. 0 I am not particularly pessimistic or discouraged about the future.

   1 I feel discouraged about the future.

   2a I feel I have nothing to look forward to.

   2b I feel that I won't ever get over my troubles.

   3 I feel that the future is hopeless and that things cannot improve.

H. 0 I don't feel I am any worse than anybody else.
   1 I am critical of myself for my weaknesses or mistakes.
   2 I blame myself for my faults.
   3 I blame myself for everything bad that happens.

Processing the data

There is a major difference between self-report questionnaires and interview-based instruments in the way a diagnosis is derived from the answers. The PSE data are processed by a computer program which incorporates an algorithm, or set of rules. These assign greater weight to some symptoms than to others and attempt to reproduce the decisions a clinician makes in arriving at a diagnosis. A program of this nature not only standardises the process of diagnosis, which varies considerably from one psychiatrist to another, it makes the rules open to examination. By comparing the diagnoses of individual psychiatrists with the output of the program and discussing the differences, the diagnostic rules used by clinicians (which often remain unformulated) can be brought into the open and studied. As we shall see later, the opportunity to make this comparison internationally revealed striking differences between the Russians, the Americans, and the rest of the world in the rules governing the diagnosis of schizophrenia.

The answers to self-report questionnaires are dealt with in a much simpler manner. The scores on each question are simply added up to give a total score, and if this exceeds a certain threshold, the person is deemed to be suffering from a psychiatric illness. We can ask whether it is legitimate to add a score of two on depression to a score of three on hopelessness and come up with a meaningful five. Are we not giving equal weight to pigs and cows? Although this objection cannot be dismissed and should give rise to a continual sense of unease about the summing of scores on such questionnaires, this has become the standard way of deciding who is suitable for a trial of treatments for depression. The use of a 'Hamilton score' of fourteen or above has been the criterion for selection of patients for many internationally recognised studies, funded by prestigious scientific bodies. Furthermore, changes in such total scores have been used regularly to decide whether one treatment is more effective than another. The expression of the patient's experience in numbers, however spurious in principle, has been forced on psychiatric researchers by the absence of laboratory measures of mental ill-health.

Measuring stress

If the measurement of psychiatric symptoms is contentious, how much more so are attempts to quantify stress in the person's environment. One of the first instruments was developed in 1967 by Thomas Holmes and Richard Rahe,[9] whose interest was aroused by the high proportion of men who developed a psychiatric illness shortly after joining the American navy. They compiled a list of what they called Life Events, which were sudden happenings in a person's life which would be expected to have a psychological impact. There are events that we would all think worthy of inclusion, such as losing your job or the birth of a baby, but then there are hard choices over less portentous happenings, such as finding that someone has scraped your parked car. Faced with the problem of determining the relative impact of their list of events, Holmes and Rahe decided to rely on the common sense of the ordinary citizen and asked a panel of nearly 400 non-professional people to rank forty-three events in order of severity. They were advised to base their judgement on the intensity of response and the time required to adjust one's accustomed pattern of life to the event. There was generally good agreement between the judges on the rank order, with death of spouse heading the list, followed by divorce, and with Christmas coming one from last.

Life events and schizophrenia

Ground-breaking as Holmes' and Rahe's innovation was, there are faults with the method that were picked up by George Brown, a British sociologist who has made many creative contributions to the field of social research in psychiatry.[10] Starting his research in the 1950s, he introduced three modifications which jacked up the technique to a much higher level of sophistication. Two of them aim to unravel the problem of cause and effect, which we shall encounter again and again in these pages. If a life event is to be a potential cause of a psychiatric illness, it is obvious that there has to be a time interval between its occurrence and the beginning of the illness. However few psychiatric illnesses develop abruptly over a few days, and some individuals experience a year or more of gradually deteriorating health before the illness declares itself with characteristic symptoms. Some people who eventually arrive at the clinic with schizophrenia have endured many months of poor concentration, sleeplessness and irritability, symptoms which in themselves are not diagnostic of any psychiatric illness. Nevertheless, these heralds of illness may so impair people's ability to work that they may be dismissed from their job.

William left school at eighteen and found a temporary office job in a software firm. He did well for the first six months and was being considered for a permanent position. However, he began to experience difficulty getting up in the morning and started arriving late. When he was reprimanded by his manager he argued fiercely, claiming that it was not his fault. He was given a warning and for a week or so his timekeeping improved. Then it was discovered that work he was supposed to have completed was left undone. He was dismissed and stayed at home, spending most of the day in bed. A few weeks later he started to complain that people were following him in the street and that his bedroom was bugged.

In this example, losing the job was not a cause of the illness but followed from the problems William experienced through its early manifestations. To clarify this confusion, Brown stipulated that in studies of life events only patients with a clear-cut onset of illness should be included, and furthermore that the onset should be dated conservatively, that is as far back in time as suggested by the history of its development. In addition he distinguished between events that had clearly been brought about by the patient's behaviour (dependent events), those that *might* have been so caused (possibly independent events), and events that could not be ascribed to any action of the patient (independent events). Returning to Shakespeare's list of events from *The Comedy of Errors*, the first two, loss of wealth through shipwreck and death of a friend, are obviously independent events, while the third, an extramarital affair, would be classified as a possibly independent event or a dependent event according to the nature of the illness. For instance, some patients who develop mania (a state of excitement) become promiscuous during the early phase of the illness. Brown excluded dependent events from consideration and conducted separate analyses for independent and possibly independent events. His first study to introduce these innovations was conducted on schizophrenia with the collaboration of Jim Birley, a psychiatrist. They used a sample of employees from a south London factory as a control group and found that fourteen per cent of them experienced an independent life event in any three-week period before the date of the interview. The patients had a similar rate in each three-week period covered by the interview except for the one immediately preceding the onset of an episode of schizophrenia, when the proportion with an independent event rose to forty-six per cent. This clustering of events in the three weeks before an attack of schizophrenia strongly suggests that a proportion of such attacks (nearly a third) are brought on by the stress of a life event.

Life events and depression

Brown next turned his attention to depression, but was still not entirely satisfied with the measurement technique he was using. From his research on schizophrenia he had learned that the same event could have a very different impact on people depending on their life circumstances. For example, the reaction to the death of a parent would depend on one's relationship with the deceased person, as well as their age at death, the nature of their terminal illness, and the time period over which they died. He was not convinced of the value of Holmes' and Rahe's panel of ordinary citizens for this purpose, and instead introduced a method of assessing what he termed the 'contextual threat' of particular events.[11] His data indicated that the events preceding a depressive illness represented the loss of a valued relationship, a cherished goal, or a material object of value. In order to assess the psychological implications of such an event for particular individuals, it is necessary to know a great deal about their life and the nature of their relationships with the significant people in their social ambit. In collaboration with Tirril Harris, Brown developed an interview schedule to collect this information; the Life Events and Difficulties Schedule (LEDS). Armed with these data, a group of researchers meet to discuss the meaning of each event in the context of the person's life circumstances and to reach a consensus on the level of severity it represents. After receiving training, researchers can reach a high degree of reliability in making these judgements.

The innovative nature of this technique needs to be seen against the tendency to collect increasingly larger samples of subjects, which is occurring throughout medical research. The greater the number of subjects, the higher the likelihood that the researcher will obtain a result that can be shown to be important by statistical tests. As sample sizes increase, it becomes more and more difficult to collect detailed information about each subject, so that researchers are always seeking short cuts to obtain data. Hence the popularity of self-report questionnaires over in-depth interviews. As a result of this trend, the uniqueness of the individual becomes sub-merged in the ocean of extensive, but not intensive, data. Brown has shown that it is possible to retain a focus on the individual subject even when collecting quite large popu-lation samples.

Vulnerable women

Brown's and Harris's research was focused on women, since population surveys regularly show that women are almost twice as likely as men to develop depression. They studied population samples in London and used the PSE to determine which women were currently suffering from depression. By comparing non-depressed with depressed women, they were able to show that the latter experienced an excess of mod-erately or severely threatening life events in the three months before the onset of their symptoms. Brown and Harris not only provided research evidence for the popular belief that stress can bring on depression, but went on to identify factors that made particular women more vulnerable to life events than others. Some women in their sample experienced threat-ening life events without developing depression during the next three months. By comparing these subjects with the depressed women, Brown and Harris picked out three factors making women particularly likely to develop depression fol-lowing a stressful life event: loss of the woman's mother before she was eleven years old; three children under the age of five years; and the absence of an intimate relationship with a partner. Each of these vulnerability factors has different social and psychological implications, although they may be linked in interesting ways.

Michael Rutter,[12] a child psychiatrist who worked with George Brown in the 1960s, conducted a comprehensive review of the research on separation from one's mother and came to the conclusion that separation was not inevitably harmful to mental health. The effects depended on whether there was a reasonable mother substitute available in the form of other relatives or foster parents, or whether the child was consigned to the not-so-tender mercies of institutional care. Subsequent to Rutter's review, it has become known that physical and sexual abuse have been horrifyingly common in British children's homes. It is likely that girls who have lost their mother and have not experienced adequate substitute care, fail to value themselves as women. It is also known that abuse in childhood damages a person's self-image. Low self-esteem has been found to characterise people with depression, and could also lead to choosing a partner who fails to provide emotional support. Women who have been abused as children often form relationships with men who are likely to repeat the abuse. The stressful nature of caring for three children under the age of five is self-evident; however, we should take account of the influence of social class on this factor. Working-class women are less likely to be able to plan the interval between their children than middle-class women, while the latter have more resources to buy in help with child care. By an 'intimate' relationship, Brown and Harris meant one in which the woman could confide in her partner and receive emotional support. For most subjects intimate relationships were with male sexual partners, but some women achieved intimacy and received emotional support from other women in a non-sexual relationship.

Support for these findings came from a large-scale survey in the north west of England in 1998. Judy Harrison and her colleagues in Manchester sent out Goldberg's General Health Questionnaire to 61,000 adults and received completed forms back from sixty-three per cent, the usual level of response to postal surveys.[13] A high score on the questionnaire indicates that the person is suffering from depression or anxiety. The strongest association with a high score was not having someone to talk to about problems. Contact with a friend in the previous two weeks was linked with lower scores. I will return to the importance of these confiding friendships later.

The research of Brown and Harris has become justly famous for identifying social factors as making both remote and recent contributions to the causation of depression. How do these findings square with biochemical theories? They are, of course, not mutually contradictory. The fact that SSRIs, working on neurotransmitters in the brain, can relieve depression does not negate the influence of social factors in bringing about and perpetuating the condition. I will present research bringing together these disparate perspectives in Chapter 4.

Neurasthenia in China

A thorny problem affecting the clinical management of depression is the strong tendency for the symptoms to recur. For this reason, many experts recommend taking antidepressant drugs for at least six months, and some stipulate one year. But what if the social circumstances contributing to the depression have not altered when the patient stops the medication? An intriguing study in China illuminates this question. Arthur Kleinman,[14] an American anthropologist and psychiatrist, became interested in the diagnosis of neurasthenia, regularly used in China but no longer found in the diagnostic vocabulary of psychiatrists in the rest of the world. He interviewed a consecutive series of one hundred patients who attended the psychiatric outpatient clinic of a hospital in Hunan for the first time, and who were given the diagnosis of neurasthenia. As he had anticipated, he found that ninety-three of the hundred patients satisfied the criteria of the American diagnostic system for a depressive illness, although only nine of these complained of depression. The great majority presented exclusively or predominantly with bodily symptoms, a phenomenon I will return to in Chapter 6. Kleinman then treated the depressed patients with antidepressants, following which sixty-five per cent reported that they were substantially improved six weeks later, and another seventeen per cent that they were slightly improved. However, thirty per cent considered their social impairment to be worse, and thirty-seven per cent sought further help from practitioners of traditional Chinese medicine and from Western-style doctors. Kleinman concluded, 'Medical treatment for chronic conditions without significant psychosocial intervention exerts only a limited effect on the overall illness.' He recommended that psychiatrists should direct their efforts to changing the patient's social environment, including interventions on a large scale. While psychiatrists' power is puny compared with the forces behind the Chinese Cultural Revolution, altering the patient's immediate social environment would be feasible. In Chapter 3 we describe the effects of such social engineering on a micro scale.

Manic-depressive illness

Depression varies considerably in severity, ranging from the relatively mild varieties that Brown and Harris studied in community samples, to a degree of intensity where people may be so slowed down in thought and action that they are unable to move or speak. At this severe end of the spectrum patients may develop delusions and hallucinations, symptoms that are commonly seen in schizophrenia and are described in detail in Chapter 2. The severe type of depression is also associated with mania, its opposite in terms of speedy thinking, talking and moving. There have been long and inconclusive arguments in the psychiatric literature as to whether the depression that is part of manic-depressive illness lies on a continuum with milder forms, common in the community, or whether it should be classified as a distinct condition. Once again, psychiatric diagnosis founders on the absence of characteristic laboratory findings. What has been established, however, is that manic-depressive illness runs in

families and that it is strongly determined by heredity. It
has been argued that psychiatric conditions with a strong
inherited basis are largely attributable to biochemical changes
in the brain. At its most extreme, this stance has been sat-
irised as 'the crooked gene gives rise to the crooked thought'.
The argument can be extended to propose that strongly
inherited conditions are less influenced by factors in the
social environment. Depression with delusions and hallucinations is one of the rarer psychotic illnesses, and so far
the role of life events in determining its onset has not been
established. Mania has been more extensively studied in this
aspect and several researchers, including myself, have found
that independent life events cluster in the few weeks before
the first onset of this illness. Interestingly, one study found
that there was no excess of life events preceding later episodes
of mania. This suggests that life events play an important
role in setting the illness in motion, but it then develops a
momentum of its own, perhaps driven by biochemical
changes in the brain, and uninfluenced by environmental
stress.

One other aspect of manic-depressive illness marks it off
from the milder form of depression, and that is the response of
the symptoms to a naturally occurring salt, lithium chloride.
Many patients find that their mood swings, both up and down,
are controlled by taking lithium chloride. Once again this
was a serendipitous discovery. Lithium chloride, which has a
salty taste, was used as a substitute for table salt (sodium
chloride) for patients with high blood pressure who needed to
restrict their intake of sodium. It was noticed that hyper-
tensive patients on lithium chloride were more stable in
mood than those not using it, and it was tried out for patients
with mania and found to be effective.

The measurement of depression

I have described the range of disturbances of mood from mild forms of emotional distress to manic-depressive illness and have shown how psychiatric researchers have attempted to identify when depression should be treated. This has been done by using a combination of a qualitative approach, exploring the person's experience of mood changes, and a quantitative approach, adding up scores on a list of symptoms. No doubt mistakes are made either side of the boundary between distress and depression, but in the present state of knowledge this is the best practical solution. To return to the example which opens this chapter, if Andrew had been given a questionnaire to fill in, his score could have been used to decide whether he was suffering from a depressive illness. However, although this would be the procedure for a research study, it would certainly not be used by his general practitioner, who would rely on clinical skills to make the decision. Unfortunately it has been well established that general practitioners miss one-third of the cases of depression that come to their clinics. This is not a trivial problem since even the milder forms of depression can disrupt the person's life and relationships, an issue to which I will return later.

At the end of this chapter I referred to manic-depressive illness, one of the psychoses. In the next chapter I will explore how psychiatrists distinguish between this illness and schizophrenia, the other major psychosis, and investigate the cultural and political forces that shape the process of diagnosis.

Chapter 2 | Moscow and Washington versus the Rest of the World

Delusions and religious beliefs

In the previous chapter I emphasised the importance of thoroughly exploring the patient's experience in order to determine which types of symptoms are present. In no area of symptoms is this more important than those characterising the psychoses. The term 'psychosis' is used for conditions in which the patient loses touch with reality; these include manic-depressive illness and schizophrenia. Up to the end of the nineteenth century these were lumped together under a general category of 'madness'. It was the German psychiatrist Emil Kraepelin who separated off the two entities in 1896, naming them 'manic-depressive psychosis' and 'dementia praecox'. In 1911 Eugen Bleuler, a Swiss psychiatrist, coined the term 'schizophrenia', which has displaced Kraepelin's original label. The symptoms that the two psychotic conditions have in common are delusions and hallucinations. Delusions are defined as false beliefs, which are not shared by others from the person's cultural background, and which cannot be shaken by argument. The proviso about the cultural background is essential but gives rise to many difficulties in interpretation.

Particular problems arise in relation to religious beliefs. The beliefs of mainstream religions which have millions of adherents create no dilemmas, but small sects can raise the difficult issue of what constitutes an acceptable belief. Two recent examples are the sect headed by Jim Jones in Guyana and the Branch Davidian sect in Waco, Texas, led by David Koresh. Both ended tragically: Jim Jones' group of more than 700 followers committed suicide at his instigation, while most of Koresh's group died in a fire when their headquarters were stormed by federal troops. When a large group of people share a set of beliefs, however unusual they may seem to outsiders, they form a subculture which legitimises their convictions and invalidates their being labelled as delusions. An even more extreme example was the suicide of a small group of people in America and Switzerland as the comet Hale–Bopp passed close to the Earth. These people believed that they would be transported by aliens as the comet passed by and that they had to quit their earthly bodies in order to achieve this. This last example raises the question of how large a group has to be before it forms a recognisable sub-culture. The Hale–Bopp group of about two dozen people was probably close to the lower limit of size.

The complicating factor is that groups holding very unusual beliefs attract people who are deluded and who may find shelter in such a group, at least for a while. There is evidence that Jim Jones believed that he was the new saviour and that he had special powers of healing. He must have been convincing and plausible to have accumulated a large band of followers who accepted his claims, and were willing to die for him. There have been other historical figures who have claimed to be the Messiah: Shabbetai Zvi in Turkey during the seventeenth century persuaded a large number of his fellow Jews that he would lead them to Jerusalem to re-establish the land of Israel. When threatened with death by the sultan he converted to Islam. Since the eighteenth century no more false Messiahs have emerged from among the Jews, as western peoples have become increasingly sceptical about the religious claims of individuals. Joan of Arc would not be able to persuade the French army to follow her into battle today on the grounds that she heard angelic voices giving her commands. At the time, the English soldiers who captured her did not dispute that she heard spirit voices, but they identified their source as the Devil rather than God, and burned her as a witch. While we no longer deal with witches so barbarically, they have not disappeared from our culture. There are groups of people practising as witches in Britain today and following satanic rituals. It should be evident that in order to judge the status of a person's belief, it is necessary to be familiar with the convictions of any subculture to which the patient belongs. In the multicultural societies of today in which many small sects flourish, no individual could be expected to be familiar with all the subcultures likely to be encountered. In the absence of the necessary understanding of a subculture, it is essential to interview a person from the same cultural group as the patient, usually a relative, in order to learn about their shared beliefs.

Hallucinations and bereavement

Hallucinations, the other characteristic symptom of psychotic illnesses, are perceptions without a stimulus in the external world. The most common form is hearing voices in the absence of any person, but hallucinations can occur in any of the other senses – vision, touch, smell and taste. Hallucinations should not automatically be considered an indication of a mental illness. Half the people who have been recently bereaved see or feel the loved person after their death.

Betty's husband died suddenly after a brief illness. They had been married for over thirty years and she felt very lonely without him. Shortly after he died she began to see an image of him sitting in his favourite chair when she entered their lounge. He was dressed in his customary clothes and appeared to be watching television although the set was not on. She was about to say something to him when she remembered that he was dead, and the image vanished. She continued to see his image for a number of years and found it comforting rather than eerie.

Some bereaved people feel the warm body of their former partner lying beside them in bed. Occasionally people who have been very close to a pet animal see or hear it after it has died. One young woman told me that after her dog died she would hear it scratching at the door to be let in. So real was this sound to her that she was impelled to go to the door and open it. These experiences can persist for years, but are rarely recounted to other people because of the fear of being thought mad. Since such a high proportion of the population is affected, this type of hallucination cannot be taken as a sign of illness.

Hallucinations in healthy people

There exist traditional cultures in which it is considered a privilege to hear the voices of ancestors. A person who returns from the forest and tells other villagers about this experience is certainly not thought of as mad. There are also cultures where hallucinatory experiences are actively sought, usually as part of a religious ritual and often by eating hallucinogenic plants, for example the peyote cactus in South America. Where hallucinations are valued by the culture, it is possible that people are more likely to report them, or, more interestingly, have a lower threshold for experiencing them. Probably we all have the capacity to hallucinate under certain circumstances. In the 1960s there was a flurry of research into the effects of sensory deprivation following the 'brainwashing' of captured American soldiers during the Korean war. In fact my own research career began with an experiment on sensory deprivation. I did not have access to resources to fit out a sophisticated laboratory, so I improvised with bits and pieces of equipment. I used army surplus goggles with writing paper in front of the lenses to obscure any definite images. The subjects also wore headphones through which I played 'white noise' – the kind of hissing sound that a badly tuned radio makes – and gloves made from sheets of foam rubber, and during the experiment reclined in an adjustable chair in a quiet room. I used volunteer medical students for this experiment. Even with the crude equipment I had constructed, half of them developed hallucinations during the three hours in the room, some of them within a few minutes of starting. One subject reported the following experiences:

> I just got an image of a head and shoulders then, of a man. I think he's wearing a suit 'cos there's clean outlines to his shoulders ... I got a strange vision then. Someone with a white robe. Like a knight with a white coronet. It was very vivid ... Saw a hunchback then. Saw him then as an image as if he was standing twenty feet away ... It's like looking up at a ceiling now. I can see the join between the ceiling and the walls. It's a long box-like room, relatively very high.

In the 1970s Mary Schwab conducted a survey of the general population in northern Florida.[15] She asked respondents: 'How often do you see or hear things that other people don't think are there?' She found that young people were much more likely to report hallucinations than the middle-aged, but this could simply have been due to their use of street drugs. Black respondents were twice as likely as whites to report hallucinations, and there was also a link with religious affiliation. The highest proportion of reports were from black Baptists, black Methodists and members of the Church of God, while the lowest were from Lutherans, Presbyterians, white Methodists, Episcopalians and Jews. The top score was reached by members of the Church of God, twenty-one per cent of whom reported hallucinations. These findings strongly suggest that certain sects encourage and even reward visionary experiences.

If delusions and hallucinations overlap with the experiences of mentally healthy people, how do we recognise that a person is suffering from a psychotic illness? The answer lies partly in the duration of the experiences and partly in their quality. The hallucinations of bereaved people fade in a few seconds, while those of the subjects in my sensory deprivation experiment lasted for a matter of minutes. People with psychotic illnesses can experience delusions and hallucinations for weeks, months or even decades. Furthermore, in the course of a psychosis, a person usually has a large variety of both delusions and hallucinations. Some of the delusions are clearly attempts to explain what is happening: if you were to suddenly start hearing voices when there was no person present, what sense do you think you would make of it? You might think at first that you were mistaken, but if it went on for hours you would have to find a way of coming to terms with it. At the beginning of these experiences, patients often consider a variety of explanations, including the possibility that they are going mad. This is, of course, very frightening to contemplate, so they usually settle on an explanation that is tolerable. I once looked after a general practitioner who had developed a psychosis. Somehow he was able to retain a professional stance towards his symptoms at the same time as being immersed in the experience. He told me he was suffering from auditory hallucinations, then added in an agonising tone, 'but the voices are driving me mad'.

Explaining hallucinations

Patients need to come to an understanding of two kinds of problem: how are these unusual experiences produced, and why is it happening to them? The mode of production is chosen from the available knowledge about influences that operate over a distance. In developing cultures, spirits of the ancestors or magic are common choices, whereas in developed countries, radio waves, computers, satellites or even extra-terrestrials are cited as the origin of the voices. Even in developed countries spiritual forces still have credence, and God and the Devil feature in some patients' accounts. Explanations for why they should be chosen for these special communications tend to be either positive – they are the new Messiah, a member of the royal family, or recruited by MI5 – or negative – the IRA or the KGB are after them, or the Devil is trying to take over their mind.

Distinguishing schizophrenia from manic-depressive psychosis

We now need to return to Kraepelin's historical division of the psychoses into manic-depressive illness and the condition named by Bleuler as schizophrenia. Mania and depression are polar opposites of mood. The patient with mania is excited or even elated and feels on top of the world. Any delusions or hallucinations that develop are in keeping with this mood, so that patients believe they have been chosen by God to save the world, that they can heal the sick and foretell the future, and they hear the voices of angels praising them. Patients with a depressive psychosis believe they are the worst sinners in the world, that they have brought ruin on their families and are condemned to eternal punishment. They hear voices saying that they are evil and should die. While people with schizophrenia can become depressed or excited, their delusions and hallucinations are not in harmony with their mood. Whereas people with severe depression believe they deserve punishment, people with schizophrenia are indignant at the persecution directed at them.

In addition to this disjunction between the prevailing mood and the tenor of delusions and hallucinations, schizophrenia is characterised by a group of unusual experiences. Another German psychiatrist, Kurt Schneider, described these clearly in 1957 and proposed that they were cardinal signs of schizophrenia. He did not claim that they occurred exclusively in this condition, and studies of these first rank symptoms, as

Schneider termed them, have shown that they are occasionally shown by patients with severe depression or mania. But once again, the lack of a laboratory test for any of these conditions means that we cannot tell whether Schneider was correct in viewing his first rank symptoms as defining a central syndrome of schizophrenia. However, they are of the greatest importance to the story I am about to tell concerning international disagreements over diagnosis, so I will describe them in some detail.

One cluster of symptoms comprises four forms of interference with the normal process of thinking:

1. Patients feel that thoughts entering their mind do not belong to them and must have originated from outside.
2. Trains of thought terminate abruptly leaving nothing behind so that patients feel that their thoughts have been extracted by some outside agency.
3. The patient's thoughts seem to be transmitted to other people so that what we normally experience as a private experience becomes a public one.
4. Thoughts are immediately repeated in the same form but without the sense of volition and ownership that we take for granted. One patient described this to me as: 'I think something and then it rethinks it for me.'

A related symptom affects actions rather than thoughts. Patients no longer feel that they are in command of their own body. Movements occur without their willing them, the voice that issues from their mouth has been produced by someone else, even their feelings can seem to be imposed on them. These experiences can be so pervasive that the patient feels possessed by some other person or a spiritual entity.

One of the most common first rank symptoms is a particular form of auditory hallucination. It may take the form of a voice commenting on the patient's thoughts and actions in the third person, for example, 'He/she is going to the kitchen. He/she is sure to make a mess of things', or of two voices discussing the patient between themselves as though the person were not present.

Most of these distressing symptoms involve the disruption of a central function of the mind which is so essential to our sense of self that we take it for granted without question, namely that we are in the driving seat and have full control of our thoughts and actions. Although the workings of our unconscious reveal themselves in dreams, slips of the tongue, difficulties in recalling particular words or names, and other phenomena identified by Sigmund Freud, we never feel displaced from the centre of control to the extent to which patients with first rank symptoms do.

Theories of the causation of schizophrenia

Early in the twentieth century, clinical observers noticed that schizophrenia tended to run in families. This observation can be explained in at least two ways: there are genes that carry a susceptibility to schizophrenia; and disturbed parents drive their children mad. Theories that parents caused the illness by the way they treated their children were proposed in the USA by several groups of researchers in the 1950s and '60s, and by Ronnie Laing in Britain.[16] Steven Hirsch and I reviewed all the published work on this topic in 1975 and came to the conclusion that there was no solid evidence involving parents in the causation of schizophrenia.[17] On the other hand, research into the inheritance of schizophrenia has produced positive results. The closer the blood tie between an individual and a person with schizophrenia, the greater the risk of developing the same illness. People whose parents both suffer from schizophrenia have the highest risk, about fifty per cent. Strong evidence also comes from studies of one-egg (monozygotic) and two-egg (dizygotic) twins. For dizygotic twins, who share half their genes, if one twin has schizophrenia the other twin has a twenty per cent chance of developing the illness. For monozygotic twins, who share exactly the same genes, the equivalent risk is fifty per cent. This much higher risk for a monozygotic twin supports inheritance as a major contributor to the causes of schizophrenia. But – and this is a very big 'but' – half the twins who have the same genes as their affected twin do *not* fall ill. This proves that the environment must be playing a part in the causation of schizophrenia, although which particular aspects of the environment are involved remains uncertain, a theme that I will pick up again later.

While the evidence for a genetic contribution to schizophrenia is generally accepted, the nature of the brain problem that gives rise to the characteristic symptoms of the illness is still unknown despite increasingly sophisticated techniques of producing pictures of the brain at rest and during activity. A theory that has been popular for over forty years concerns a particular type of chemical transmitter in the brain. In Chapter 1, I described the theory that serotonin plays an important part in the origin of depression. The transmitter that was believed to be important for schizophrenia is dopamine. This chemical became the focus of interest with the introduction of the first drug that benefited patients with delusions and hallucinations, chlorpromazine (Largactil).

The story of the discovery of its value for psychiatry is yet again one of serendipity. Chlorpromazine was in use in the 1930s as an antihistamine and for clearing the urine of bacteria and the gut of worms (its trade name, Largactil, is an awful pun on 'large number of actions'). One of the standard tests of the safety of a drug is to find out what dose will kill fifty per cent of a group of laboratory mice. When it was tested in this way, the pharmacologist noticed that those mice that survived were very sleepy, and had the bright idea of trying it on psychiatric patients. It proved to be much better than a general sedative, in that it reduced the patients' delusions and hallucinations, and its use rapidly spread around the world. Chemical tests on the brain showed that it blocked the action of the transmitter dopamine on the nerve cells. Furthermore, when a whole range of similar drugs were eventually marketed, they were all found to have the same action on the brain, and their potency in improving patients' symptoms was closely related to the strength of their dopamine blocking effect. The resultant theory that an excess of dopamine in the brain was the basic problem in schizophrenia held sway for decades.

Many years ago the Wellcome Trust founded a unique club for active researchers in the field of schizophrenia, bringing together scientists from many different disciplines who would otherwise be unlikely to share ideas. At one meeting, an eminent biochemist stood up and announced that after more than ten years' work on the dopamine hypothesis, he had come to the conclusion that it was a blind alley. There was a shocked silence. It was as dramatic as if the Pope had announced that he no longer believed in God. No one commented, and this announcement had no perceptible impact on the psychiatric community's faith in the dopamine hypothesis. Since 1992, a new series of antipsychotic drugs has been introduced which are just as effective against the symptoms of schizophrenia as the older drugs but have little or no blocking action against dopamine. As a consequence the dopamine hypothesis was toppled from its pedestal, ten years after the agnostic biochemist's declaration, and as yet has not been replaced with an alternative theory.

American and British diagnoses

I described in Chapter 1 the construction of the Present State Examination (PSE), the semi-structured interview for assessing psychiatric symptoms. Schneider's first rank symptoms occupy a prominent position in the schedule because, in the set of rules used to process the PSE data, the presence of just one of them leads to a category of schizophrenia. One of the incentives to construct the PSE was the possibility of making international comparisons of diagnosis. At the end of the 1960s, Morton Kramer drew attention to the fact that the diagnosis of schizophrenia was being made twice as commonly for patients on their first admission to hospital in America as for their British equivalents.[18] If this was a true reflection of a difference in the frequency of appearance of schizophrenia, it would demand investigation of the possible causes, a situation we will encounter in the last chapter. Kramer's observation prompted a bilateral study using the PSE to assess patients on both sides of the Atlantic, and a team of psychiatrists who used the same method to make diagnoses.[19] Standardisation of these procedures eliminated the difference in frequency of the diagnosis of schizophrenia between the USA and the UK, showing that this was simply a consequence of transatlantic variations in psychiatrists' approaches to interviewing and diagnosis. The reasons for the difference revealed by this study lie in the training of the psychiatrists, in particular the domination of psychoanalysis in the USA at that time compared with its marginal position in the UK. The process by which a psychoanalytic training leads to a broad concept of schizophrenia is explained below.

An international study of diagnosis

At about the same time as this US–UK comparison began, the World Health Organisation (WHO) was planning a more ambitious study of the same nature but involving nine different countries. The aim was to collect at least a hundred patients in each centre who had been given a local diagnosis of schizophrenia and then to compare them in terms both of their symptoms as recorded with the PSE and the diagnostic categories produced by the associated computer program. Of course the set of rules incorporated in the algorithm of the computer program does not invest the resulting diagnostic categories with any absolute truth. The rules represent the consensus of the three psychiatrists who constructed the program in 1974, John Wing and John Cooper, both British, and Norman Sartorius, a Croatian.[20] They are as arbitrary as any other psychiatrists' diagnostic rules. However, the program possesses the advantage of always doing the same thing each time it is fed data from a patient, which cannot be claimed by any psychiatrist. Additionally, as stressed in the preceding chapter, because the rules are explicit they open up the possibility of studying the diagnostic procedures used by individual psychiatrists.

The centres chosen for the International Pilot Study of Schizophrenia (IPSS), as the WHO study was named, were deliberately sited in a mixture of developed and developing countries. The former comprised Aarhus (Denmark), London (UK), Moscow (then USSR), Prague (then Czechoslovakia) and Washington (USA). The developing centres were Agra (India), Cali (Colombia), Ibadan (Nigeria) and Taipei (Taiwan). I had just finished my study on sensory deprivation and had joined the Medical Research Council social psychiatry unit at the Institute of Psychiatry in London, which was one of the research centres of the IPSS. I had recently been trained by John Wing, director of the unit, to use the PSE, and I was asked to collect the cases for the London centre. Thus began my involvement with the WHO which still continues, and which took me all over the world, stimulating my interest in cultural issues as they relate to psychiatry.

Back-translation

The PSE was developed in English and had to be translated into the seven other languages used in the IPSS centres, and then back-translated. This procedure revealed some interesting problems: for instance, there was no equivalent word for 'depression' in Yoruba, the language used in Ibadan. In Chinese, only a single word could be found to stand for 'anxiety', 'tension' and 'worrying', which refer to different symptoms in the English version of the PSE. These difficulties in translation were much more common in the section dealing with neurotic symptoms than in the psychotic section, so did not impede the principal aim of comparing the diagnosis of schizophrenia across the participating centres.

The consensus and the odd ones out

The psychiatrists in each centre were required to make their own diagnosis on the patients collected by their team. They could base this on the PSE ratings and any other information they had gleaned about the patients. Their diagnoses were then compared with the categories produced by the application of the computer program to the PSE ratings. The surprising result, displayed in Table 1, was that there was a high level of agreement between the computer-generated categories and the diagnoses made by the psychiatrists in seven of the centres. The two centres showing major discrepancies between the computer categories and the local diagnoses were Moscow and Washington. If these two centres are excluded, the overall agreement between the other seven centres and the computer categories is ninety-six per cent on schizophrenia and eighty-six per cent on manic-depressive psychoses and the neuroses. Even in the two rogue centres,

Table 1 Discrepancies between computer-generated categories and psychiatrists' diagnoses in the International Pilot Study of Schizophrenia

Centre	Percentage discrepancy
Aarhus	13.8
Agra	13.1
Cali	7.0
Ibadan	9.8
London	3.9
Moscow	35.1
Prague	13.7
Taipei	4.6
Washington	21.5

there was a heavy reliance on Schneider's first rank symptoms as indicators of the diagnosis of schizophrenia. Across all nine centres, if any one of the first rank symptoms was rated as present, there was a likelihood of ninety-five per cent or greater that the psychiatrist would diagnose schizophrenia.

It is no surprise that the London psychiatrist, myself, was in closest agreement with the computerised categories, since I worked in the same institution as the main architect of these, John Wing. What does require an explanation is that the Taiwanese psychiatrists agreed almost as closely with the computer output as I did. The answer lies in some curious quirks of history. Japan occupied Taiwan following the Sino-Japanese war in 1895. Psychiatric training in Taiwan during the period of occupation was strongly influenced by the prevailing Japanese culture. Because of political and ideological links with Germany, Japanese psychiatry adopted the German approach to assessing symptoms, including Kurt Schneider's identification of first rank symptoms. In the opposite geographical direction, the German influence on British psychiatry was strengthened by refugees from Hitler's persecution. A number of Germans fled to the UK in the 1930s and became prominent and influential teachers in psychiatry and psychology. It is ironic that imperialism and persecution should have been largely responsible for the concordance reached between psychiatrists worldwide on diagnosis.

Psychoanalysis in the USA

Now we need to consider why the Washington and Muscovite psychiatrists were outliers in the international comparison. The disagreement between the Washington psychiatrists and the other centres echoed the findings of the US–UK comparison described above, but I have yet to explain the reasons behind it in detail. They lie in the domination of American psychiatry by psychoanalytic theory and practice up to the 1980s. Woody Allen's films capture the ethos of that era, when many Americans who considered themselves to be enlightened and could afford the fees, engaged in a personal analysis, regardless of whether or not they suffered from psychiatric symptoms. In response to this demand from clients for what was seen as a prestigious and health-promoting experience, the majority of psychiatrists underwent a training in psychoanalysis, involving a heavy expenditure of time and money. As a result, psychoanalytic theory dominated the assessment of patients' mental state and the diagnostic process.

Psychoanalysis places a great emphasis on unconscious mechanisms that are believed to underlie symptoms. These were proposed by Sigmund Freud and expanded by his daughter, Anna, a child psychoanalyst. They are considered to be ways in which the mind deals with threatening information and the basic drives of sex and aggression. These mechanisms include repression, pushing uncomfortable thoughts or experiences out of the mind so that they do not intrude on consciousness, and projection, attributing to other people our own characteristics that we find unacceptable. There is a relatively small number of these proposed mechanisms compared with the rich diversity of symptoms. Specific mechanisms such as projection are considered to be characteristic of psychoses. Analytically trained psychiatrists focus on identifying the unconscious mechanisms being employed by the patient rather than the precise nature of the symptoms, which are viewed as relatively superficial phenomena. This leads to a broad definition of schizophrenia, which includes most cases that would be diagnosed as mania by British psychiatrists, and a sizable proportion of those who would be identified as having a personality disorder. It must be emphasised that diagnostic practices in the USA have changed dramatically since the 1980s, partly in response to the striking findings of the US–UK comparison and the IPSS, and partly due to the spectacular decline in popularity of psychoanalysis among American psychiatrists.

The KGB and psychiatry

The reasons for the Muscovite psychiatrists being out on a limb are completely different and have sinister undertones. At the time of the IPSS, Moscow psychiatry was dominated by one man, Andrej Snezhnevsky, who was head of the Psychiatric Institute. The structure of the Institute reflected the strict hierarchical nature of Soviet society, so that all the psychiatrists employed there were constrained to use Snezhnevsky's diagnostic system. This was based, not on the nature of the symptoms, but on their time course. Any psychotic symptoms that were recurrent were taken as an indication that the illness was schizophrenia. The Muscovite psychiatrists were perfectly capable of identifying symptoms of mania and depression, but if more than one episode of any of these symptoms occurred, the diagnosis of schizophrenia was given. Thus a case history could read, 'The patient has had two episodes of mania and one of depression, and is suffering from schizophrenia.' To summarise this approach crudely, 'If you've had it before and you've got it again, it's schizophrenia.' The social adjustment of the person between episodes of illness was also given great diagnostic importance. If there were indications of difficulties in adjusting to society, this was taken as confirmatory evidence of schizophrenia. Incidentally this system had not spread to Leningrad, where the psychiatrists were making diagnoses in a similar way to the concordant IPSS centres. The Moscow approach to diagnosis led to a broad definition of schizophrenia, as in America, but for completely different reasons. It also opened the door to exploitation of psychiatry by the Soviet secret police, the KGB.

Individuals who openly protested against the Soviet system were diagnosed as harbouring 'reformist delusions'. As I have argued above, this is a misuse of the term 'delusion' since there were enough dissidents to form a substantial subculture sharing the same views. But the term was sufficient to allow the Moscow psychiatrists to make a diagnosis of psychosis (being out of touch with reality), and a person who protested on more than one occasion would inevitably be given the label of schizophrenia. This was a boon for the KGB who could then invalidate the political activity of the dissidents by locking them up in psychiatric hospitals and forcibly administering antipsychotic drugs which they did not need. It is difficult to determine whether many of the Moscow psychiatrists were actively collaborating with the KGB, but my opinion is that Snezhnevsky introduced his diagnostic system in good faith and it was then exploited politically. What is clear is that he failed to protest at what was happening to the dissidents. The Royal College of Psychiatrists of the UK, of which he was a corresponding member, initiated the process of expelling him, but before it could run its course, he resigned.

Soviet dissidents in Israel

Some years later the Soviet authorities relaxed their ban on the emigration of Soviet Jews to Israel, and among the immigrants were several dissidents who had been given a diagnosis of schizophrenia and had been incarcerated in psychiatric hospitals. I took the opportunity of a visit to Israel to interview three of these men with the PSE. They were all happy to cooperate with the procedure and to talk openly about their history. Two of the men were vigorous, high-achieving individuals who had no symptoms of psychosis when I saw them and, as far as I could determine, had never suffered from any psychiatric illness. The third man was a quiet academic of high moral principles, who had been deeply affected by the Soviet invasion of Czechoslovakia to suppress the resurgence of democracy. He resolved to commit suicide publicly as a protest and set fire to himself in a public place. His life was saved by some passers-by and he was given a diagnosis of schizophrenia and admitted to a psychiatric hospital. He had no symptoms when I interviewed him, and despite my careful questioning of him about the period before the suicide attempt, I could find no evidence of depression or any other psychiatric illness. I came to the conclusion that his action was what the sociologist Emile Durkheim identified as altruistic suicide, giving up your life for a higher cause.

Politics, economics and diagnosis in the USA

I do not want to give the impression that psychiatric diagnosis is influenced by political forces only in totalitarian countries. There have been two recent examples of this type of influence in the USA, one of which concerned the status of homosexuality. Following the revealing findings of the US–UK comparison and the IPSS, vigorous efforts were directed at compiling guidelines for diagnosis which would be accepted and used by all American psychiatrists. The resulting document is named the *Diagnostic and Statistical Manual of Mental Disorders*, and is now in its fourth edition (DSM-IV). During the preparation of a revised version of the third edition (DSM-III-R), the issue came up of whether homosexuality should remain in the *Manual* as a pathological condition. The political organisations in the United States that represent homosexual interests put pressure on the psychiatrists to end what they saw as an aspect of persecution. It is well to remember that the Nazis insisted that homosexual men wear a pink triangle, and that thousands were murdered alongside six million Jews and over 100,000 mentally ill people. The American Psychiatric Association put the matter to the vote and homosexuality ceased to be included as a disease by a majority decision.

The other example illustrates the power of commercial forces to alter diagnostic habits. In the absence of a national health service, American medicine is dominated by private health insurance agencies. These operate a system known as managed care, which gives them the power to withhold funding for treatments they consider to be ineffective. Thus they refuse to pay for days spent in hospital by patients with schizophrenia during which they receive no drug treatment. Personality disorders represent a difficult area for psychiatry, since there is no generally accepted treatment that is considered to work. This is a problem facing the current British government in attempting to formulate a new Mental Health Act. Personality disorders are excluded from compulsory admission under the existing Act of 1983 as they are not considered to be amenable to treatment. For the same reason, the health insurance agencies in the USA were unwilling to fund psychiatric care for people with a personality disorder.

Before the 1980s a diagnosis termed 'multiple personality disorder' was very rarely used. In 1973 an American psychiatrist, Cornelia Wilbur, published an account of a case of hers in a book titled *Sybil*, which was made into a successful film. The fame achieved by this single case study was followed by a great increase in the professional use of the diagnosis. In 1980 multiple personality disorder became an official diagnosis incorporated in the third edition of the *Diagnostic and Statistical Manual* (DSM-III), although the term was changed to 'dissociative identity disorder' for DSM-IV in 1994. Ian Hacking records that by 1992 there were hundreds of patients with multiple personality disorder in treatment in every sizable town in North America, and that entire private hospitals dedicated to the illness were being established all over the continent.[21] Hacking points out that doctors treating this condition must capture as much insurance coverage for non-drug treatments as possible. At the ninth meeting of the International Society for the Study of Multiple Personality and Dissociation in 1992, the conference theme was health insurance. The result of the official recognition of the condition by its inclusion in the DSM is that health dollars can now be claimed for the treatment of this personality disorder. It is striking that this diagnosis is rarely made in Europe, and it is not included in the European equivalent of the DSM, the

International Classification of Diseases (ICD-10), compiled
by the World Health Organisation.

The frequency of appearance of schizophrenia across cultures

Social, political and commercial forces could not influence
the diagnostic process if there were objective tests for diagnostic entities. In their absence, the reader could be excused
for taking a nihilistic view of the attempts by psychiatrists to
classify diseases. However, it is necessary to retain a sense of
perspective on the issue. Seven out of the nine centres in the
IPSS reached a close agreement on what symptoms constituted a schizophrenic illness. This engendered sufficient
confidence in the mental health division of WHO, directed
by Norman Sartorius, to proceed to the next step in their
ambitious programme, an international study of the frequency of appearance of schizophrenia.

Incidence and prevalence

Here I need to introduce two technical terms, incidence and
prevalence, and explain how they differ. *Incidence* refers to
the number of people who first develop an illness over a set
period of time, usually one year. *Prevalence* includes anyone
who is ill at the time of the head count, which is a mixture
of new cases and people who have been ill for some time.
Prevalence can be measured at a single point in time, the
point prevalence, or over a year, the annual prevalence. If
you are interested in studying the causes of illness, it is the
incidence rate that is important. When the incidence varies
between two populations, one can look for other differences
between the two groups that might explain this variation.
One of the first studies of this kind was carried out in London
during the nineteenth century by John Snow to investigate
the causes of a cholera epidemic. By plotting the number of

new cases (the incidence rate) on a map of London, he discovered that households supplied with water from one reach
of the Thames, below a sewage outlet, were much more likely
to develop cases of cholera than households that received
their water from a reach of the Thames above the sewage
outlet. By removing the handle from the Broad Street pump,
distributing water from the lower reaches, he halted the epidemic.

The principal aim of the second WHO study was to
measure the incidence of schizophrenia in centres that differed widely in their social, economic and cultural aspects,
thus providing a greater opportunity to identify the possible
causes of the illness. Twelve centres were chosen in developed
and developing countries, and in urban and rural settings.
The study was named the Determinants of Outcome of Severe
Mental Disorders (DOSMD) since a second aim was to
compare the outcome for patients in the various centres. This
was prompted by the results of a follow-up of patients in the
IPSS, which showed that patients in developing centres had
a better outcome than those from developed centres. This
was surprising because, of course, psychiatric facilities were
much sparser in the developing centres so that patients
received much less professional care. The interpretation of
this finding was clouded by the fact that the IPSS sample
contained both first-onset cases and patients who first became
ill some years back, and that the mix of these was different
between centres. To make a true comparison of outcome it
was necessary to confine the samples to first-onset cases only.

Making contact with the services

It is actually almost impossible to pick up people at the first
onset of symptoms of schizophrenia, because they do not
immediately seek professional help. In fact the average time
lag between onset of symptoms and making the first contact
with medical services is well over a year, and is considerably

longer for men than for women. In practical terms, then, the DOSMD study recorded first contact with medical services for psychotic symptoms. This is not too demanding an exercise when services are centralised in a hospital, but becomes increasingly difficult with the dispersion of services throughout the community. In a developing country there is the added complication of limited resources of Western type and the consequent flourishing of traditional forms of treatment. Hence, in the developing countries, the researchers had to identify all the traditional healers in the area of the survey, and gain their cooperation in notifying the research team when they saw suitable clients. The difficulties of this endeavour are such that in only one developing centre, Chandigarh in north India, was the finding of cases considered tight enough to provide a reasonably reliable estimate of the incidence of schizophrenia. This is a pity, since the greatest contrast in socio-economic conditions and culture was between developed and developing countries. At least Chandigarh included both an urban and a rural environment.

The centre in north India

The city of Chandigarh was built from scratch on an agricultural plain as the intended shared capital of two adjoining states, Punjab and Haryana. However, Punjab took it over exclusively, which remains a bone of contention between the two states. It was designed by the French architect, Le Corbusier, and contains many striking public buildings, including a Postgraduate Medical Institute. The city has attracted highly educated people to live there, so that during the period of the DOSMD study, the literacy rate was seventy per cent. There could hardly be a greater gulf between the lifestyles in the city and in the surrounding rural area, where people live in houses built of mud bricks and thatched with straw, the social unit is the extended family, and the literacy rate at the time was thirty per cent. Traditional healers were the main source of help for mental illnesses, but the psych-iatry department at the Postgraduate Medical Institute, headed by Professor Narendra Wig, set up a mobile team which visited the villages in rotation to hold outpatient clinics and to facilitate the aims of the research.

Variations in incidence across centres

Twelve centres were originally included in the DOSMD study, but checks on the completeness of case-finding cast doubt on the procedures in four of the centres, which were consequently excluded from the analysis. The centres in which few patients were considered to have slipped through the net were Aarhus, Chandigarh (urban and rural), Dublin, Honolulu, Moscow, Nagasaki and Nottingham. As in the IPSS, the translated version of the PSE was used in each centre and the local psychiatrists were trained to interview patients and rate their symptoms reliably. The ratings from the PSE were processed using the associated computer program. In view of the central role played by Schneider's first rank symptoms in the diagnosis of schizophrenia across countries, incidence rates were calculated for two types of schizophrenia, with (S) or without (non-S) first rank symp-toms. The number of cases of each type was divided by the number of people in the population studied who were between the ages of fifteen and fifty-four, since this was the age range of patients accepted into the study. The results are displayed in Figure 1.

It is evident that there is much less variation in the inci-dence of S schizophrenia than in the incidence of the non-S variety. The first contact rate for S schizophrenia ranged from 7 cases per 100,000 population per year in Aarhus to 14 per 100,000 in Nottingham. A statistical test showed that a difference this small could have occurred by chance, so that the rates from the eight centres should be treated as equal. This is an extraordinary result, since no other disease occurs

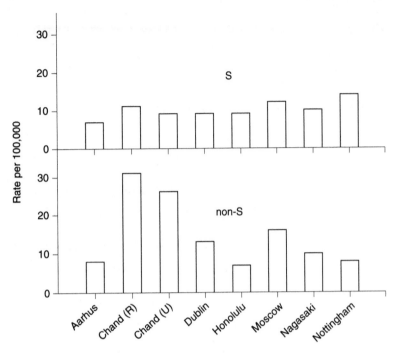

Figure 1 Incidence rates for schizophrenia with (S) or without (non-S) Schneiderian first rank symptoms. Chand (R), rural area of Chandigarh; Chand (U), urban area of Chandigarh

with the same frequency around the world. It suggests that environmental factors play little part in the causation of S schizophrenia, otherwise the contrasting social, economic and cultural environments of the centres would have led to large variations in the incidence.

Some critics have objected to the method used in this international study, claiming that the PSE acts like a grid imposed on the rich variety of unusual mental experiences represented by the patients in the different cultural settings. The psychiatrists using the PSE only pick up what is considered to be abnormal in the Western countries in which it was developed. An appropriate analogy would be a chip machine: whatever shape the potatoes are that go into the machine, they all come out as chips. This argument has some validity, but its force is weakened when we examine the incidence rates of non-S schizophrenia. These provide a very different picture, with a range from 7 per 100,000 in Honolulu to 31 per 100,000 in the rural area of Chandigarh. A more than fourfold difference of this magnitude must be taken seriously and points to the importance of environmental factors in the causation of this type of schizophrenia. The different balance of causative factors in S and non-S schizophrenia constitutes an argument for considering them to be distinct diseases. This is not a revolutionary idea: when Bleuler first introduced the term, he named the condition 'the group of schizophrenias', implying that it covered more than one disease. The resolution of this issue will have to await the discovery of underlying biological abnormalities which might distinguish the component diseases. In the meantime, the DOSMD findings illustrate how an epidemiological study can raise questions about accepted diagnostic concepts. Studies of this nature can also suggest possible causes of diseases but cannot prove a causal connection. This requires an intervention, such as John Snow's removal of the handle of the Broad Street pump to halt the cholera epidemic. In the next chapter I will describe how interventions can be used to establish causes of psychiatric conditions.

Chapter 3

The Human Probe

Cause and effect

When two events happen very closely together in time we tend to assume that the earlier event caused the later one. Whether assumptions of causality are based on previous experience or are 'hard-wired' into the brain is not known for certain, although Jean Piaget, a Swiss psychologist, demonstrated that children start to make these assumptions when they reach a certain age. While they prove to be correct most of the time, it is possible to make mistakes, as we saw in unfolding the story of life events. The point can be illustrated by the 'Spot the Ball' competition. Faced with a snapshot of footballers in a variety of positions and postures, from which the ball has been erased, the competitor has to guess the location of the ball. The fact that there are few winners shows how difficult this task is. If you were shown a videotape of the thirty seconds of preceding play, from which the ball had also been deleted, it would be much easier to locate the ball in the still image. Research into human behaviour faces the same problems. A cross-sectional study is equivalent to the snapshot: it can establish connections between events but cannot tell which is the cause and which the effect. A study conducted over a period of time contributes more to our understanding of causality, but there are strict limits to the length of time a study can take. These are partly imposed by

the availability of funds and partly by the needs of researchers
to obtain publishable results and move on to the next experiment. The longest study I have been involved in lasted thir-
teen years and was a five-year follow-up of nearly 700 patients
who had been discharged from two psychiatric hospitals over
the course of eight years. I had to seek renewal of my funding
every three years and often did not know until the eleventh
hour whether or not the study was going to continue. A major
problem with psychiatric research is that the time period of
interest is the lifespan of the patient. We would dearly like to
know how experiences in childhood shape the susceptibility
of the adult to psychiatric illnesses, and how this is affected
by the changes in the life cycle all the way through to old age.
No single researcher can encompass the entire life of his or
her subjects, but there are ingenious short cuts. Lee Robins,[22]
an American researcher, was interested to discover what happened in adult life to children who showed disturbed behaviour. In 1966 she looked backwards in time to records of
children who had been referred to child guidance clinics in
the 1930s. She was able to trace many of these children who
had become adults by the time she began her study. This
strategy enabled her to link disturbances in childhood,
recorded by the staff of the clinics, with psychiatric problems
in adulthood. Useful as this method of condensing time was,
Robins was restricted to what the clinic staff thought important to record more than twenty years earlier.

Humans looking at humans

It is not only the dimension of time that is problematic for
the researcher into human behaviour, it is also the fact that
the experimenter and subjects occupy the same space. We
have no difficulty in being objective about things that are
astronomically bigger than us, such as stars, or micro-
scopically smaller, like viruses. In fact we can only study
them by using instruments which bring them closer to our

own size. The problem with human beings as objects of study is that they are the same dimensions as the researcher, they occupy the same space, and we are biologically and culturally primed to react to people in specific ways. We have developed techniques that increase the distance between ourselves and the people we study. We can focus on a small part of the person; in the case of the brain, making records of its electrical activity or images of its structure. We can use audiotapes or videotapes, which we can stop and start at will, and play slower or faster than they were recorded, thereby altering our time relationship to the subjects. But however this distancing is achieved, eventually what has been learned has to be integrated into an understanding of the person as a whole living being. I write 'has to', but not all scientists feel this as an imperative. Many are more comfortable with visualising the person as a collection of chemical systems, or of strands of DNA. This has led to the charge of scientific reductionism: reducing the person to a series of formulae which maintain the distance between researcher and subject in the service of objectivity. What is lost by this manoeuvre is the exquisite sensitivity we possess to other people's feelings and behaviour, which is essential for the functioning of humans as social beings. I shall now describe one of the most innovative techniques in psychiatric research, which instead of rejecting our subjectivity, capitalises on this very sensitivity to other people in order to measure their feelings.

Out of the asylums

The spur to the development of this measurement technique was the change in attitude to the care of psychiatric patients in the old asylums. Patients who had spent many years of their life in a psychiatric hospital were discharged to live in the community. It has been claimed that this was a direct consequence of the introduction to psychiatry of chlorpromazine (Largactil, *see above*), which controlled delusions and hallucinations. However, chlorpromazine came into use for this purpose in 1955, whereas some hospitals, such as Mapperley in Nottingham, began to reduce their number of beds in the late 1940s. The first wave of patients to be resettled during the 1950s were in relatively good shape, and went to live with their families or in private accommodation with landlords or landladies. Sadly, after a time some of them had to return to the asylum when they fell ill again. This prompted George Brown and colleagues, working in the social psychiatry unit at the Institute of Psychiatry in London, to follow up a group of discharged patients to investigate what might account for their failure to remain in their new homes.[23] The unexpected finding was that patients who returned to live with their parents were more often readmitted than those who resided with brothers or sisters, or in private lodgings. George Brown followed a hunch that it was the emotional interaction between patients and their parents that led to a return of their illness. Before pursuing this line of enquiry he had to overcome a major obstacle: no measure of emotional interactions between people existed. To understand how this extraordinary deficiency persisted through more than fifty years of psychological studies, I need to make a brief excursion into history.

The split in psychology

From its beginnings, psychology developed along two paths which became increasingly divergent. The path beaten by Freud and his followers began with introspection, an attempt to establish the workings of the mind by reflecting on your own thoughts and feelings. Freud analysed his own dreams, and caught himself out in slips of the tongue and other actions he had not intended. In his writings he sometimes presented his discoveries as though they related to a patient of his, when they were actually a product of self-analysis. This was partly to protect the most intimate aspects of himself, but undoubtedly also to give a more 'objective' appearance to his discoveries. Following Freud, psychoanalysts use their own knowledge and experience of feelings and drives to understand the patient's emotions and behaviour. They convey their understanding to the patient in the form of an interpretation, which is a reformulation of the patient's speech, or silences, in terms of the patient's relationship with the analyst. This is based on the assumption that the patient behaves towards the analyst, an unknown stranger, as though the analyst were one of the salient figures in the patient's life – a process known as transference. Freud recognised that the analyst also develops emotional responses to the patient, referred to as countertransference, which he saw as an obstacle to the process of therapy. However, in 1950 Paula Heimann introduced the idea that analysts could use their feelings towards the patient to further their understanding of the patient's emotional state, since the patient made an important contribution to these feelings.[24] Her insight introduced greater reciprocity into what had been a somewhat one-sided relationship.

The other path was taken by psychologists who were determined to shape their discipline into a science. The stress was on objective measurement, large samples of subjects, and reproducible results. Many of the experiments were conducted on animals, usually rats, but occasionally monkeys, with very limited application to the understanding of human emotions. One school of psychologists, the behaviourists, was formed in the early part of the twentieth century. Led by Watson and Skinner in the USA, they rejected the idea of studying thoughts and feelings and strictly confined their observations to forms of behaviour. They decided to treat the human mind as a 'black box' with unknowable contents, and only attempted to measure the inputs and outputs. The barrenness of this approach led to a crisis in psychology in the 1960s, with a dawning realisation that the apparent objectivity might be alright for the study of rats, but was spurious for humans since the researcher could never be invisible to the subjects. Even if the experimenter were not present in the room, the subjects were well aware that someone had set up the experiment and would be evaluating the results. Hence their reactions were bound to be influenced by their emotional response to the testing situation and the absent researcher; which the psychoanalyst would recognise as transference. It was considered preferable to acknowledge these responses openly and to view them as contributing to the data yielded by the experiment. Psychologists began to appreciate the value of single-case experiments, which involved the intensive study of one subject, often using qualitative measures. While in this way experimental psychology began to approach psychoanalysis, there was very little prospect of a meeting of minds since psychoanalysts seemed unable to contemplate the measurement of the unconscious and dynamic forces with which they wrestled daily. At just this time the problem of integrating the subjective and the objective was solved by the development of a measurement technique which became known as 'expressed emotion'.

Measuring relatives' emotional responses

Measurement of expressed emotion was the brainchild of George Brown and Michael Rutter, both of whom we encountered in Chapter 1. It took them several years to finalise the technique, which centres on an interview with a relative who is caring for the sick person. Initially, in the 1960s, the research concerned people with schizophrenia, but it has now been successfully applied to a wide variety of psychiatric and physical illnesses. The interviewer asks the carer about the patient's symptoms and behaviour in the previous three months, a subject most carers will talk about eagerly. The interview, which occupies up to one and a half hours, is audiotaped. No ratings are attempted during the interview, but are made when the interviewer can listen to the recording

at leisure. This entails going over a crucial sections several
times in order to be confident of the assessment, so that rating
can take up to twice as long as giving the interview and is
obviously a painstaking procedure. The rater listens carefully
not only to what the relative says, but also to the way in
which the words are spoken. The rater treats the relative's
voice as a channel of information about the relative's emotional attitude to the patient. To make this clear I am going
to ask you to conduct a little experiment. Try saying as calmly
as possible, 'My son lies in bed till the afternoon, and when
he gets up he doesn't wash himself.' Now repeat exactly the
same words, but convey as much anger with your voice as
you can. If you think about how you changed the emotional
tone of the sentence, you will find that the second time, you
probably spoke louder and faster, and there were more ups
and downs in the pitch of your voice. These clues from the
voice, along with the content of speech, are used to identify
the emotions expressed by the relative. In this example what
is rated is termed a 'critical comment' and the number of such
comments made in the course of the interview is counted.

The principle of the technique is that the rater's own emotional response to the relative's utterances is used to identify
the emotion the relative is expressing. There is an obvious
parallel with the psychoanalyst's use of countertransference,
except that analysts do not discuss with each other the clues
they use to identify particular emotions in their patients: this
ability is taken for granted as common to all human beings.
But in a research project it is essential that the experimenters
are equally sensitive to these clues. Therefore they have to
attend a two-week training course in interviewing and rating,
during which the techniques are explicitly discussed and a
number of master tapes are rated. Trainees have to reach a
high level of agreement on rating the master tapes before they
gain approval to do their own studies.

Criticism and hostility

Critical comments are the core element in the expressed emotion (EE) ratings, being the most commonly encountered. The number of such comments made in the interview is counted and indicates how angry the relative feels about the patient. In British studies, about one-third of relatives of patients with schizophrenia make no critical remarks, showing a high degree of tolerance for the difficulties of living with such a person. The average number of critical comments is around six, so this is used as the threshold to divide relatives into high- and low-criticism groups. At the extreme upper end of the range a few relatives manage a machine-gun rate of fifty to sixty in an hour. An extreme form of criticism is rated as 'hostility', which is recognised either as a bunching of critical comments or a critical attitude towards the patient as a person, rather than confining the remarks to the patient's behaviour. Comments such as, 'She's the laziest girl you've ever met' would rate as hostility.

Overinvolvement

The third component of EE is overinvolvement, which comprises a number of different behaviours and attitudes. Overprotectiveness is shown by relatives who behave towards the patients as though they were much younger than their actual age. Thus one mother would not let her daughter aged twenty cross the road on her own, while another bathed her son who was in his late teens. Some relatives become overemotional in the interview, weeping and making dramatic statements such as, 'I feel her illness has ruined my life.' In judging whether excessive emotion is being shown, the rater has to take account of the circumstances of the carer, including the cultural background. Women show their emotions more readily than men, and people from Mediterranean countries are more expressive than Scandinavians. I once asked a

Spanish colleague how he recognised overinvolved carers. He replied that he called them 'butcher relatives', and in response to my incomprehension explained that these were people who said, 'If it would make my son well, I would cut off my arm and leg.' Giving due consideration to the influence of the carers' culture is built into the training course, which often includes trainees from many different countries and cultures. The fact that sensitivity to cultural variations is integral to the measurement technique has enabled it to be used successfully in China, Japan and India as well as across Europe and America. Two additional aspects of overinvolvement are excessive self-sacrifice, when relatives devote too much of their time and emotional energy to the care of the patient at the expense of their own needs, and symbiosis. This term, borrowed from biology, refers to two organisms from different species which are mutually dependent on each other for survival, such as cleaner fish on the coral reef and their client fish whom they rid of parasites. The human pair also exhibit a lack of psychological boundaries, the carer believing that she or he understands the thoughts, feelings and needs of the patient without having to be told. While partners can be just as critical of patients as parents can, overinvolvement is rarely seen in partners and is much more common in mothers than in fathers.

Expressed emotion and the course of schizophrenia

When high levels of critical comments or overinvolvement are expressed, or hostility is present, the carer is denoted as 'high EE'. George Brown and his colleagues, Jim Birley and John Wing, first used this measure in 1972 in a study of patients with schizophrenia.[25] It proved to be remarkably successful in distinguishing patients who did well from those who did poorly. Relapse was defined as a return of the symptoms of schizophrenia in those who had completely recovered, or an intensification of symptoms in those who had never been completely free of them. More than half the patients who lived with high-EE relatives relapsed in the nine months after returning home from hospital, whereas only about one in six of those in low-EE homes did so.

A patient of mine, Sarah, lived with her elderly parents who were very conventional. Sarah was quite rebellious and upset her father who regarded himself as a pillar of the community. One day Sarah came home having dyed her brown hair bright red. Her father was appalled and had a furious row with her in which he criticised her appearance and behaviour, and called her a slut. She went to her room to escape his anger and within half an hour began to hear the critical voices which had been a feature of her previous attack of schizophrenia.

The dramatic difference in outcome between patients in high-EE and low-EE households appeared to explain the findings of the original study of patients discharged from the asylums; but was it a fluke? The essence of scientific experiments is replicability: can a different group of researchers in another place using a new sample of subjects produce the same results? There are so many extraneous factors that cannot be controlled, particularly when studying people, that replication is essential to prove that the original findings were not due to these uncontrolled factors. Consequently, at the beginning of the 1970s Christine Vaughn and I undertook a replication study.[26] Although we were working in the same unit in which the original study was done, George Brown and Jim Birley had left, and we collected a completely new sample of patients and their relatives. Both of us were trained to rate EE by the original researchers, and became highly reliable at doing this. The training has now been formalised as a course that is run regularly and is attended by trainees from all over the world. Almost all of them learn to make reliable ratings in two weeks, evidence of the applicability of the technique across languages and cultures.

Protection from a high-EE relative

In addition to repeating the design of the previous study, we decided to include a group of patients suffering from depression. The question we were addressing was whether the link between EE and course of illness was limited to schizophrenia, or whether it might apply to other psychiatric conditions. We chose to focus on depression because it provides such a contrast with schizophrenia, and for this reason we excluded any depressed people who were experiencing delusions or hallucinations. The part of our study dealing with schizophrenia turned out to be an almost perfect replication of the earlier research: exactly half of our patients in high-EE homes relapsed over nine months, compared with only twelve per cent of those living with low-EE relatives. The figures for the earlier study were fifty-eight per cent and sixteen per cent. Since we used the same measuring instruments for all aspects of our study as in the previous work, we felt justified in pooling the data from the two studies, which amounted to well over one hundred patients. This was a large enough group to carry out some more detailed analyses. We confirmed a finding from the earlier study that patients living in high-EE homes had two ways of protecting themselves from relapse: either by taking antipsychotic medication long-term, or by keeping out of the relative's way. Patients who spent little time with their high-EE relative were much less likely to relapse than those who were constantly with them. The protective effect of low social contact was as powerful as taking maintenance medication. If patients both took medication and kept a low profile there was an additive effect, resulting in a relapse rate of only fifteen per cent, which is close to that of patients in low-EE homes. The remarkable aspect of this finding is that a pharmacological agent and a form of social behaviour can act together to reduce the likelihood of another attack of schizophrenia. The challenge we faced was to formulate the susceptibility to schizophrenia in such a way that it could accommodate the influence of factors in two such different domains.

Expressed emotion and the course of depression

Before grappling with that problem we need to consider the findings for the depressed patients. Firstly they differed from the patients with schizophrenia in their living situations: whereas less than half of those with schizophrenia lived with a partner, virtually everyone with depression did so. As already mentioned, overinvolved attitudes are virtually confined to parents, so that they were not a feature of the relatives of the depressed patients. Among these carers, critical attitudes loomed large; in fact they turned out to be every bit as critical of their partners as were the relatives of the schizophrenic patients. However, when we applied the threshold of six critical comments that had worked with schizophrenia, it failed to separate patients who stayed well from those who suffered a return of depression. We looked carefully at the data and found that by lowering the threshold to two critical comments we could distinguish patients who did well from those who did poorly. This means that depressed people are even more sensitive to criticism from their relatives than are people with schizophrenia. This indication of the importance of the relationship with a partner in perpetuating depression accords with the identification by Brown and Harris of a lack of a supportive relationship as one of the vulnerability factors for developing depression in response to a life event (see Chapter 1).

Expressed emotion and schizophrenia: opposing models

It is tempting to interpret these results as proving that disturbed relationships make both schizophrenia and depression worse, but this inference cannot be made from snapshot studies of this kind, because of the problem of determining

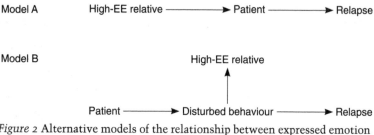

Figure 2 Alternative models of the relationship between expressed emotion (EE) and relapse of schizophrenia

the direction of cause and effect, which I have already discussed. We can usefully examine the alternative interpretations of the link between EE and the course of schizophrenia.

In Figure 2, model A presents the 'common sense' interpretation that the relatives' critical and overinvolved attitudes have a direct psychological impact on the patient causing a return of schizophrenic symptoms. Model B, which is equally plausible, postulates that the patient's disturbed behaviour provokes the relatives to develop high-EE attitudes, and eventually develops into a full-blown schizophrenic attack. In this model there is no direct link between EE and relapse of the schizophrenic illness. In fact, in both the studies I have described, the degree of disturbed behaviour was measured with just this possible scenario in mind. In neither study was there any link between the level of disturbed behaviour and the relatives' EE rating. Low-EE relatives appeared to be able to tolerate quite a severe degree of disturbance without becoming critical or overinvolved. Unfortunately this does not resolve the issue. Any characteristic of the patient which may not even have been measured, could both provoke high-EE attitudes and render the patient more likely to relapse. It is here that a video film of the family recorded over a prolonged period would throw light on this problem. We could watch changes in the behaviour of the patient and the carers and decide which came first in time. But that strategy is impractical because we could never record family life unobtrusively, although it has been attempted for television programmes. Even more daunting is the prospect of analysing months of videotapes, considering that it takes many times as long to analyse such material as it does to record it. The answer lies elsewhere – in the form of the human probe.

Probing the family system

We can think of the family as a system. Observed from the outside, it is so complex that it is very difficult to appreciate the way it functions. Many attempts have been made to measure what goes on in families, but at best they capture only glimpses of the complexity. But suppose the observer enters the system and tries to change it from the inside. The family has to react to the presence of a foreign body in its midst and in doing so reveals many of the strategies it employs to maintain the integrity of the system. For example, various members of the family will try to form an exclusive alliance with the stranger in order to bolster their authority in any power struggle. Some may take advantage of the apparent safety guaranteed by the stranger to air grievances that have remained unspoken. Others may try to incorporate the intruder into the family and behave towards her or him in the way they would treat a particular family member.

In order to tackle the 'cause or effect' problem I have presented in respect to EE and the course of schizophrenia, I decided that the most telling strategy was to introduce a human probe into the families. I shall call this person the therapist, since the ultimate goal was to improve the outcome for people with schizophrenia. I certainly do not mean to imply that families caring for someone with this condition need therapy. When a family member develops schizophrenia, it taxes the resources of the family mightily. The remarkable fact is that half the families in Britain faced with this challenge respond with low-EE coping behaviours, managing to avoid becoming angry or overinvolved with the patient. High-

EE relatives are not sick and do not need treatment, but, for one reason or another, are using coping strategies that actually make things worse, and need to be helped to employ more effective ways of dealing with the daily problems that schizophrenia generates. The changes that the therapists were attempting to achieve were clearly definable: to reduce EE from high to low, or to reduce social contact between patient and high-EE relative from high to low. But how was this to be done?

Trials and placebos

In 1976 I assembled a team of colleagues to work out how to achieve these changes, and then to put the ideas into practice as therapists. They were Elizabeth Kuipers, a psychologist who already had experience of working with families with a behavioural approach, and two psychiatrists with a psychoanalytic approach, Rosemarie Eberlein-Fries and David Sturgeon. We spent some months deciding on the constituents of our intervention and then jumped in at the deep end. What we had put together was a combination of education about schizophrenia, teaching the family how to tackle problems and to improve communication, methods of decreasing anger and overinvolvement and of resolving conflicts, strategies for reducing contact, and a focus on developing realistic expectations for the patients. We did not have an overarching theory of family function but were like magpies, taking bits and pieces from different schools of therapy which we thought might help us succeed in our aims. To convey an idea of our approach, I will give an account of how we intended to reduce the output of critical comments. As I have already explained, critical comments are an expression of the relative's anger. Relatives get angry with patients because they care about them. If you didn't care for a person, their behaviour would be a matter of indifference to you. Therefore we bring out the caring attitude behind the anger. For example:

Mr Brown, referring to his son, Daniel, in an angry tone of voice: He's always wearing a dirty shirt.

Therapist: You really care about your son's appearance.

Mr Brown: Of course I do.

Therapist: Would you tell Daniel how you would like him to dress?

Mr Brown: Daniel, I'd like you to wear a clean shirt.

The last communication from Mr Brown is a positive request for change instead of an angry attack, and offers Daniel the opportunity to please his father.

In order to test the value of what we were about to do with families, we set up what is known as a randomised, controlled trial. This has become the standard experimental design for evaluating new drugs and other types of physical treatment, such as surgery. Patients are assigned to two or more different treatments by a random procedure. In the dark ages before computers this was achieved by tossing a coin. Nowadays computers are used to generate sequences of random numbers. Often, the treatment under investigation is tested against a placebo, since many medical conditions can improve, at least temporarily, in response to the attention received by patients taking part in a trial. This demonstrates the powerful effect of the person's state of mind on bodily ailments, and understandably an even greater influence can be observed on psychiatric conditions. For example, patients with depressive symptoms respond better to green pills, while patients with symptoms of anxiety show a greater improvement on yellow pills, even when they contain identical medication. A study conducted in Alabama found that responses to the colours of pills varied between ethnic groups. White subjects tended to assume that white capsules were painkillers, while black subjects saw them as stimulants.

An abortive trial of psychosurgery

In the case of a drug it is easy to prepare a placebo pill which looks exactly the same but contains an inactive substance like chalk, or a placebo injection which consists only of salt water. For social and psychological treatments it is impossible to invent a placebo. In any contact between two human beings, it is not possible for one of them, the therapist, to do nothing, and any interaction, however low-key, has the potential of being therapeutic. Therefore instead of using a placebo, it is necessary to include a comparison treatment which is considered to be the best therapy in current use. Even this design is not feasible for some procedures, for example psychosurgery. Many years ago I was asked by the Medical Research Council to work with two colleagues and a group of neurosurgeons to design a trial of psychosurgery. Lobotomy, as it was originally called, was introduced for the treatment of schizophrenia in the 1930s by Egaz Moniz, for which he received one of the only two Nobel prizes ever awarded in psychiatry. Psychosurgery is no longer used for schizophrenia but is seen as an 'end of the line' treatment for patients with severe depression or obsessions who have failed to respond to anything else. It would have been unethical to subject patients to the full sequence of neurosurgical procedures with the exception of the final cut into the brain, so a placebo control was rejected. We could not employ a comparison treatment because these patients had tried everything else that might have helped. The only practical design was to use a waiting-list control; that is, patients would be randomly assigned to receive psychosurgery immediately on referral or to wait a further six months, after which they would undergo the operation. The six-month period while waiting would then be compared with the six months following psychosurgery for the experimental group. Unfortunately the neurosurgeons would not accept this design, arguing that by the time patients were referred to them, they were desperate, so the operation could not be delayed since it undoubtedly helped them. Of course no one can state this with certainty, but so strong was their investment in the procedure that the trial was not carried out, and as far as I know never has been, so that the value of psychosurgery remains untested.

Evaluating the family intervention

The design we chose for our trial was to compare our newly constructed family intervention against the usual treatment given to patients with schizophrenia, which at that time did not involve any contact with family members. We realised that at the end of the trial if our intervention proved superior to the usual treatment, we would not know whether this was simply the response of relatives to the interest shown by the therapists rather than to the particular things we were doing with them. We would then have to design another trial to sort out that problem (which we did).

We decided to conduct the trial on the patients who were most likely to relapse, because that would give us the greatest leeway to show an effect of our intervention. We selected patients who were in high social contact with high-EE relatives, knowing that even on regular medication they would have a fifty per cent chance of relapsing over nine months. We aimed to establish them all on antipsychotic medication, since it was well established by my own drug trial and by many others subsequently, that medication gave at least partial protection against relapse. The question we wished to answer was whether changing the family environment could add any benefit over and above the effect of medication. Our previous research suggested that if we could lower EE or social contact, and these were not simply byproducts of the patient's behaviour, the expected relapse rate would be around fifteen per cent.

It took five years to complete the trial and we had to wait that long in suspense to discover the answer. The first result we were intensely curious about was whether our crafted intervention had succeeded in inducing changes in the families. To our surprise and delight we discovered that three-quarters of the experimental families had reduced their EE and/or social contact levels below the target thresholds. However, forty per cent of the control families, who had received no professional help, also achieved these changes, showing that some families possess a self-healing capacity. The next question was whether these changes in family attitudes and behaviour reduced the patients' susceptibility to relapse. Half the control patients relapsed over nine months, exactly the rate we had predicted from the earlier work. For the experimental patients, rather than the fifteen per cent we had optimistically aimed at, the rate was remarkably low at eight per cent. Thus the results support the model postulating that relatives' emotional attitudes and behaviour towards the patients have a direct impact on their liability to relapse, and if these are ameliorated the course of schizophrenia can be changed. In the process of trying to establish the direction of cause and effect, we had invented a new treatment for schizophrenia.

This result was not just a flash in the pan. Numerous similar trials by colleagues in Britain, America, China and Japan have produced the same findings: that working with the families of schizophrenic patients improves the outcome of the illness. Whatever the biological basis of schizophrenia turns out to be, this body of work demonstrates that patients with this condition are extremely sensitive to the emotional environment surrounding them. In this respect they are no different from the rest of humanity, but the popular stereotype of madness (of which more later in the book) has set them apart as alien beings.

Expressed emotion and psychiatric and bodily illnesses

Some relatives have reacted negatively to these findings, feeling that they are being blamed for causing the illness, but there are a number of considerations that should reconcile them to the results. Work on EE has developed in several different directions. The measure has been applied to a wide range of psychiatric and bodily illnesses, and high levels of EE have been found in almost all of them. However, while EE has been linked to the outcome of many psychiatric conditions, including manic-depressive psychosis, eating disorders, alcohol abuse and post-traumatic stress disorder, the only bodily illnesses this relationship has been found in so far are diabetes and epilepsy. A group of American researchers has shown that people with diabetes living with a critical relative have poorer control of their blood sugar levels than those in low-EE households. However, two British teams have failed to replicate this finding. A study of children with epilepsy carried out in Britain found that children with poorly controlled epilepsy were much more likely to live with high-EE parents than children whose epilepsy was well controlled. The pervasiveness of high-EE attitudes across such a variety of illnesses argues that they cannot be a specific cause of schizophrenia, even though they may aggravate the condition once it is established. Moving in another direction, EE has been measured in professional carers working in sheltered homes, many of which have been set up for patients discharged from the old psychiatric hospitals. These homes are often ordinary houses, and, unlike hospital wards, staff and patients spend much of the day in intimate social contact, sharing household chores. In this respect, the atmosphere is much more like that in a family home, and indeed the staff commonly develop high-EE attitudes towards their charges. Several studies, including one of our own, have detected highly critical attitudes from the staff, although they do not seem to become overinvolved with the residents. The commonality of high-EE attitudes in both unpaid and professional carers and across many different disorders suggests that they are by no means an abnormal response to the demands of coping with long-term or relapsing conditions. However, once a link is established between EE and the course of an illness, a window of opportunity opens for the development of an intervention which may improve the outcome for patients. In the next chapter I will recount how we exploited this opportunity for patients suffering from depression.

Chapter 4

A Couple of Pills or Couple Therapy?

Developing and testing the family interventions for schizophrenia absorbed the energies of the research team for well over ten years. But all along I had the nagging feeling that the work on depression was a loose end that had been left dangling. I was not confident that we had established the correct threshold for critical comments, since we had simply adjusted it down from six to two by eye (so to speak), to produce a significant difference in relapse rates between the two groups of depressed patients. Consequently I was relieved when I heard in 1983 that a young graduate psychologist from Oxford, Jill Hooley,[27] was keen to try to replicate our findings for her PhD thesis. As it turned out, her results were almost identical to ours, bolstering our confidence in the cut-off point of two critical comments that we had established. Further support came from a surprising source: in 1994 Ahmed Okasha,[28] professor of psychiatry in Cairo, repeated the work with a sample of Egyptian patients and their spouses. This time it appeared that a threshold of seven critical comments gave the best separation between depressed patients with a good and a poor outcome, but there was still a significant difference between the groups using our cut-off point. The accumulation of evidence for a relationship between the partner's critical attitude and the course of depression seemed to me sufficient to take the next step of designing an intervention study. We were well into the study by 1997 when we were informed of a failure to replicate this relationship by an experienced research group in Cambridge headed by Eugene Paykel.[29] The only possible explanation we could envisage for this divergent result was that the Cambridge sample, unlike the others, contained a high proportion of middle-class women. It is conceivable that their access to material resources enabled them to compensate for the deficiencies in their marital relationship. Whatever the correct explanation for this anomalous finding, even if it had come to our notice earlier, I don't think it would have deterred us from pushing ahead with the trial of intervention. In the body of work on EE and schizophrenia, there are also some studies which failed to replicate the association with outcome, but they constitute a small minority.

Research on people differs from experiments with inanimate matter in that it is possible to gain only partial control over the conditions of the experiment. Given a constant atmospheric pressure, water uncontaminated by other chemicals will always turn to steam at the same temperature, whereas individuals vary considerably over time in the amount of provocation needed before they lose their temper. Uncontrolled factors can produce differences in results that are beyond the ingenuity of the researchers to explain. Hence, in human research the scientist is always weighing up the balance of evidence for and against a proposition, and the most convincing conclusions can be drawn when the same study has been repeated by many different teams working in a variety of countries.

Self-esteem and cognitive therapy

In designing the trial we were mindful of two streams of research in addition to the work on EE. One was the line of enquiry that George Brown had continued to pursue since identifying the vulnerability factors for depressed women. He had reached the conclusion that the central problem in depression was low self-esteem, which led women (he did not include men in his samples) to feel bereft when events occurred that robbed them of relationships or roles which helped them to establish their worth. To investigate these ideas he had developed measures of both positive and negative self-esteem. The research on EE and depression seemed to fit neatly with these notions, since being faced with constant criticism from your partner must surely lower your self-esteem unless you are very resilient. The other area of relevance was the burgeoning of non-drug treatments for depression over the previous decade. The most rigorously tested was cognitive therapy, invented by Aaron Beck in Philadelphia. This embodies a psychological approach to improving a person's self-esteem by encouraging them to question their assumptions about themselves and their abilities relative to other people. It may sound simple-minded, but part of its effect is achieved through the relationship that develops between the therapist and the patient, as in all 'talking cures' (Freud's term for psychoanalysis). Seen from today's perspective, they might better be called 'relationship therapies' since the transference (see Chapter 3) of the patient to the therapist is a vital ingredient in them all. Cognitive therapy has been tested against antidepressant drugs in numerous randomised, controlled trials, and has generally been found to be equally effective in relieving depression, and in some studies in preventing relapses.

In addition we found that there had been a handful of trials of marital therapy, which were of particular interest to us since we were planning to involve the patients' partners in the treatment. These studies, although not as convincing as the body of evidence for the value of cognitive therapy, suggested that marital therapy could also achieve an improvement in depression equivalent to that conferred by medication. Not surprisingly, it appeared that marital therapy was better than drugs at improving the couple's relationship.

Systemic therapy

In order to stabilise people with schizophrenia, it is obvious
from a compendium of trials that it is essential to use antipsychotic medication as a foundation on which family interventions are built as an adjunct. The situation is completely
different with depression, since psychological treatments
such as cognitive therapy have proved to be at least as effective
as antidepressant drugs. Therefore we felt we could take the
risk of comparing couple therapy without any added medication against the best possible course of drugs. To be accepted
for the trial, patients had to be in a steady relationship with
a heterosexual partner, and the partner had to make two or
more critical comments when given the EE interview. Only
a handful of partners made just one critical remark or none
at all. In the previous studies, researchers also found that
low-EE partners constituted a small minority, so that most
depressed patients in a relationship are exposed to criticism
from their mates. For our studies of schizophrenia, my colleagues and I developed the intervention for families, but in
order to devise an intervention for depressed patients and
their partners we called on the expertise of two systemic
family therapists, Eia Asen and Elsa Jones. At this point I
need to explain the concept behind systemic therapy.

By now the term 'ecosystem' has become part of the language: it implies that all living things are dependent on one
another and on the non-living environment for their existence. The ecosystem is thought of as maintaining a har-
monious balance which humans are disturbing by their
'unnatural' activities. A system is recognised by virtue of
having defined boundaries and of maintaining its integrity
within those boundaries. This is achieved by the existence of
feedback loops which signal when a disturbance occurs in the
system, setting in motion some compensatory action. This
attempts to correct the disturbance and return the system
to its previous balanced state. Systemic therapists view the

family as just such a system. Each family has its own boundary, although in traditional cultures the boundary may encompass several dozen people. Some years ago, during a visit to India, I stayed with a Muslim family which comprised thirty-five people living in the same household. Within its boundary the family tries to maintain stability by compensating for changes. Using as an example the reaction of the family to a therapist coming to their home (*see* Chapter 3), they may try to neutralise the perturbation caused by the therapist by socialising their relationship: asking personal questions and offering food and drink. Alternatively, they may close ranks and expel the therapist as being too threatening to their system.

A colleague and I worked with a Greek Cypriot family: a mother and her daughter who suffered from schizophrenia. The mother was very grateful for our visits and each time baked us an orange cake. We felt it would be churlish to refuse her hospitality, which also stemmed from her cultural background, so after being given gargantuan portions on our first visit, the next time we asked her to cut us each one thin slice: an attempt to set limits on her generosity. However, she was not to be confined in this way and, despite our protests, wrapped up the rest of the cake for us to take home at the end of the session.

The designated patient

Whereas doctors usually assume that any disturbance is limited to the individual who comes to them for help, systemic therapists view the family system as selecting one of its members as the 'patient' to convey a message to the source of help that all is not well with the family. Hence they call the person who presents to the doctor the 'designated patient' and turn their attention to the whole family. There are clearly limitations to this approach. When the presenting condition has a strong basis in heredity, as with Huntington's disease, it is worse than useless to treat the patient as a harbinger of the family's own disturbance, even though the relatives may well be very distressed by the appearance of the symptoms. The same considerations apply to schizophrenia, albeit that the role of inheritance is not nearly as pronounced as in Huntington's disease. The weaker the evidence for a biological determinant for the condition, the more likely it is that a systemic approach will achieve improvement in the symptoms. Thus behavioural problems in children, such as bed-wetting and school refusal, respond well to systemic family therapy.

Writing a treatment manual

We asked the two therapists who agreed to work with the couples in the trial to write down what techniques they were going to use, and to include an outline of how the therapy would proceed over the twelve to twenty sessions within which they would try to achieve their aims. They were not comfortable with this demand at first, since therapists like to feel free to follow their intuition. However, we needed them to produce a manual so that if their therapy proved to be successful, other researchers could put it to the test. I have emphasised several times the importance of replicating the findings of research on people. They did eventually provide what we wanted; a document that opens with a general statement of their approach to depression, from which it is worth quoting directly. 'Close relationships are regarded as both influencing and being influenced by the depressed patients and the symptoms. The responses of family members to the patient may be seen as helping to maintain, or contributing to the patient's distress and symptoms.' Their remedies for this situation include helping the couple to gain new perspectives on the presenting problem, to attach different meanings to the depressive behaviours, and to experiment with new ways of interacting with each other that do not include the depressive symptoms. Rather than teaching the couple how to improve their relationship, the therapists encourage them to find their own solutions so that they gain a sense of mastery over the problems.

The trial of couple therapy versus drug treatment

Preventing relapse

One of the most daunting problems posed by depression is that even when complete recovery has occurred there is a high risk of the symptoms returning. This has shaped the policy on prescribing antidepressant drugs, which is to maintain the patient on a moderate dose for at least six months after the illness has resolved. But if depression is a response to adverse social circumstances, including lack of support or constant criticism from a partner, unless these have improved, taking the person off the drugs exposes them to risk of a further relapse. I described in Chapter 1 the experience of Arthur Kleinman with victims of the Chinese Cultural Revolution, which perfectly illustrates this dilemma. Consequently, we were as interested in the potential of the treatments under study to prevent relapse as in their ability to remove the symptoms of depression. Patients were randomly assigned to couple therapy or to antidepressants. If they ended up in the latter group they were first prescribed one of the older type of drugs, known chemically as tricyclic antidepressants. If they did not respond in six weeks they were prescribed fluoxetine (Prozac). Medication was continued for one year and then stopped gradually. The patients were then followed up after a further year to test the preventive effect of the treatment. The couple therapy occupied the first nine months, following which no further treatment was offered in the period up to the two-year follow-up.

The depressed partner

During the initial assessment, not only did we measure the intensity of the patients' depression, but we asked the partners to fill in a questionnaire about their own mental health. To our surprise, one-third of the partners were suffering from depressive symptoms severe enough to need treatment. If these partners had approached us instead of the patients we would have included them in the trial as cases and considered the actual patients as partners. If both partners are equally depressed, what determines which of them presents their complaints to the doctor? The answer to this intriguing question will have to wait for a future study, but the systemic concept of the 'designated patient' appears to be entirely appropriate to at least one-third of our sample.

Dropping out of treatment

A researcher always hopes that the subjects will be well behaved in a trial, accepting the treatment to which they have been assigned and turning up for follow-up assessments. Unfortunately real life is not like that, and subjects often rebel against the artificial constraints of a controlled comparison of treatments. In this instance, even though the patients were clearly informed that the treatment they would receive was determined by chance, just over half of those randomly assigned to antidepressant drugs refused to take them or simply stopped coming to the clinic. This was not such a surprise since previous trials of antidepressants had also lost a high proportion of patients. Numerous surveys of public opinion about psychiatric treatments have shown that there is a strong feeling against antidepressant drugs, which most people believe are addictive, as explained in Chapter 1. Whatever the reason for rejecting drugs for depression, the great majority of the public favour talking cures for the whole range of psychiatric conditions. It was not unexpected, therefore, that only a small proportion (fifteen per cent) of patients dropped out of couple therapy.

Outcome of the trial

Following the period of treatment, patients were assessed again for the severity of depression. Both treatments gave considerable relief from the symptoms, but the improvement was greater for those receiving couple therapy. At the end of the second year, during which no treatment was given, the patients in the couple therapy group were still doing better than those who had been given drugs.[30] This shows that couple therapy was superior to drugs both for treating depression and for preventing the return of symptoms. This result gives support to the theory that depression is maintained by a problematic relationship between the two partners and that working to improve the relationship gives more lasting benefit than taking an antidepressant drug. It also backs up the view that depression in one partner signals a disturbance in the family system.

The value of a friend

During the mid-1990s, while our team was assessing the value of couple therapy, George Brown had arrived at a similar point in his research on the causes of depression in women. Having found that the absence of a confiding relationship increased the likelihood of a woman becoming depressed following a life event, he decide to test the effect of providing women with a befriender. Like our team, he also mounted a randomised, controlled trial to evaluate this intervention. For the study he chose women who had been depressed for at least a year, and randomly assigned them either to have a befriender immediately or to wait for one year before being offered this form of help. This type of design is known as a waiting-list control. Nearly two-thirds of the women were in a partnership, and the same proportion were experiencing severe difficulties in their personal relationships. The befrienders, all women, were recruited through advertisements in the local press, churches and health centres. They received three days' training in acting as a 'friend', listening, and 'being there' for the depressed woman.

How acceptable was the offer of a befriender? Of the forty-three women in the experimental group, twenty-five (fifty-eight per cent) engaged with the befriender, eight (nineteen per cent) refused after one meeting, and the remaining ten saw a social worker but not a befriender. It appears that the befriending service was not much more welcome than antidepressant drugs for this group of women with long-standing depression. However, at the end of a year sixty-three per cent of the women in the befriending group were relieved of their depression compared with only thirty-nine per cent of control women.[31] There was no comparison with drugs in this trial, but it shows that providing a supportive relationship for women who do not have one relieves depression. It is therefore an alternative approach to improving an existing relationship.

The biochemistry of depression

What do these trials tell us about the nature of depression? The success of these non-drug therapies impels us to reappraise purely biochemical theories of depression and the claims of the pharmaceutical industry for their products. As I explained in Chapter 1, the newest class of antidepressants, the SSRIs, increase the amount of serotonin in the brain and this is assumed to account for their effect on depression. Several other classes of drugs with actions on different neuro-transmitters, such as the tricyclics, also increase serotonin activity in the brain, as does electroconvulsive therapy. However, the effect that treatment has on serotonin activity is not directly related to the improvement in depression. No single theory of the underlying biochemical disturbance in depression can explain the action of these different treatments, but since each of them outperforms placebo, the chemical and electrical events they produce in the brain are likely to be related to the biochemical basis of depression. It would be of great interest to know whether the non-drug treatments are influencing the same biochemical events through changes in the patient's psychological functioning. One study has attempted to bring together biochemical theories and the response to psychotherapy.

Steven Rose and Sarah Willis used an indirect method of measuring the level of serotonin in the brain, as it is very difficult to gain access to the chemistry of the brain in a living person. The measure they used was the amount of imipramine (a standard antidepressant) taken up by one of the constituents of the blood, the platelets, which reflects the serotonin level. They studied patients who had attended a walk-in clinic with emotional problems and had been offered psychotherapy. They matched the patients with healthy controls and carried out the same measures on both groups at the same points in time. The Hamilton Rating Scale for Depression gave an indication of the subject's intensity of depression. Before receiving psychotherapy, the patients' level of imipramine binding was about half that of the controls. As the patients' depression improved, the level rose to equal that of the control group. This result suggests that a non-drug treatment can have the same effect on brain chemistry as drugs specifically targeted on the serotonin system.

This study illustrates the difficulties of monitoring what is going on in the brain in response to environmental changes. Rose and Willis had to be content with an indirect measure of brain neurotransmitter levels. We encountered the same type of problem in trying to link environmental stress with the development of symptoms of schizophrenia. Our different approach to this knotty problem is described in the next chapter.

| # I've Got You Under My Skin

Expressed emotion and life events

The research on how stress affects the brain to produce depression is in its infancy, whereas the same issue has been more extensively studied in schizophrenia. Before describing what has been discovered, I need to weave together the stories about life events and relatives' expressed emotion (EE). Life events happen over a short period, usually no more than a few days or a week or so. In contrast, exposure to a high-EE relative can continue over months or even years. How do these short-term and long-term stresses interact? In the study of EE and schizophrenia that Christine Vaughn and I worked on together in the 1970s we included the assessment of life events introduced by George Brown.[32] We found that patients living with low-EE relatives and not taking medication had a high rate of life events: over half of them had experienced an event in the few weeks before they fell ill. However, if they lived in a high-EE home they were no more likely to have a life event happen to them in the period before an attack of schizophrenia than a well person. Our interpretation of these results is that patients living in a high-EE environment are continually exposed to stress, which builds up to the point at which they suffer a relapse of their illness. Patients cared for by low-EE relatives do not experience stress in their daily lives until an event occurs which pushes them over the edge into a psychotic state. If this formulation is correct, one would expect patients in high-EE homes to have shorter intervals between relapses than those in low-EE homes, who stay well until a life event comes along. There is support for this from a long-term study of schizophrenia carried out in the 1980s by Robin McCreadie,[33] a psychiatrist working in Scotland. He followed patients for five years and found that those in high-EE homes relapsed about once a year, while those in low-EE homes relapsed only once every three years.

Is the laboratory neutral?

What is the impact of external stress on brain function that leads to the appearance of the symptoms of schizophrenia? Unfortunately we still understand very little about the way brain functioning in mental illness differs from that in healthy people. Modern methods of scanning the areas of the brain that are most active have shown that the frontal lobes and certain other regions of the brain show less activity in people with schizophrenia, particularly when they are suffering from an attack of the illness. But this is such a general finding, and varies so much from one individual to another, that it is of little help in answering the question I have posed. There is another, more technical problem arising from the mechanics of brain scanning. It requires the subjects to lie motionless on a couch with their head inside a large cylinder. Having gone through the procedure myself, I can confirm that it is quite stressful. Indeed, some people with even mild claustrophobia cannot tolerate it. People suffering from schizophrenia can sometimes incorporate the procedure in their delusions, fearing they are going to be electrocuted or to have their brain permanently altered. This illustrates the crucial fact for all experiments on humans that the laboratory is not the neutral place most researchers take it to be. It exerts a stressful influence which varies from person to person but is ignored in favour of the comforting myth that the laboratory is a standardised setting which affects every subject in the same way.

Measuring stress from the skin

Since the focus of our research was the stressful effect of the patient's environment, it seemed much more logical to make the measurements in a situation in which we knew the stress level, rather than in a laboratory in which we did not. Hence we took the bold step of conducting the experiments in the patients' own homes. But what could we measure of any interest using portable equipment? The answer was found in the lie detector. This piece of equipment, which has become famous through its portrayal in Hollywood films, is based on the changes in the electrical conductivity of the skin that result from sweating. The salt in sweat is a good conductor of electricity, whereas dry skin is not. Even small increases in sweating over brief periods of time can be detected quite sensitively by simple equipment. A rapid rise and fall in electrical conductivity is known as a spontaneous fluctuation (SF). The number of SFs recorded during a minute is termed the SF rate and is an indication of the level of excitation of the autonomic nervous system. This system is not under conscious control and reacts to perceived threats by preparing the individual for immediate action, traditionally summed up by the phrase 'fight or flight'. The heart races, breathing speeds up, blood is pumped to the muscles, and sweating increases, anticipating the need to lose heat generated by running or fighting.

It was not too difficult to rig up a portable machine to measure skin conductance and to take it in a van to subjects' homes. The experiments were run in 1977 by a PhD student, Nick Tarrier,[34] now professor of psychology in Manchester. Since we knew from the earlier studies that contact between the high-EE relative and the patient increased the risk of relapse, we decided to record the patient's skin conductance with only the researcher in the room for fifteen minutes and then to ask the relative to join them, and to continue recording for a further fifteen minutes. Three groups of subjects were involved; patients living in a high-EE home, patients in a low-EE home, and mentally healthy controls who lived with a relative. Nick Tarrier repeated the procedure on three occasions three months apart, and on each visit he asked the subject about life events that might have occurred in the period before the recording session.

The effect of a relative

The average SF rates for each of the groups of subjects during the thirty-minute period are shown as graphs in Figure 3 for the first occasion of testing. Looking at the control group you can see that they start out at quite a high SF rate, indicating that the novel experience of being wired up to a piece of equipment in their home was arousing. However, as nothing frightening happened after the experiment began, their SF rate descended steadily throughout the thirty minutes with a brief blip at the entry of their relative. This process of adaptation by the nervous system to something unusual happening is termed 'habituation'. If we did not habituate to new sights, sounds and other stimuli, we would be in a constant state of high arousal which would be very uncomfortable. As the author James Thurber remarked about an eccentric genius in one of his short stories, 'He constantly stimulated me to the pitch of a nervous breakdown.' The graph for patients in high-EE homes is a complete contrast to the graph of the control subjects, since their SF rate remains at a high level throughout the thirty minutes with no sign of habituation. They show a dramatic response to the entry of the high-EE relative, which is significantly greater than the equivalent response of the other group of patients to their low-EE relative. For the first fifteen minutes the graphs of the two groups of patients are indistinguishable, both remaining at high levels. However, the entry of the low-EE relative into the room causes something unexpected to happen. The patients immediately start to habituate and by the end of the second

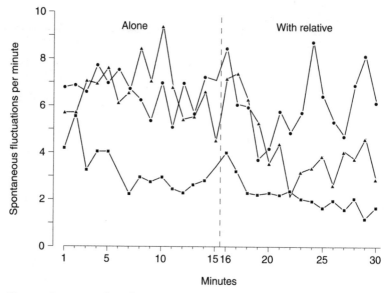

Figure 3 Mean number of spontaneous fluctuations per minute during the
test period in eleven high-EE patients (triangles), ten low-EE patients
(circles) and twenty-one control subjects (squares)

fifteen minutes are approaching the low level of the control
subjects.

This surprising finding completely changed our way of thinking about low-EE relatives. It showed that their presence was
reassuring for the patients, enabling them to come to terms
with the psychologically disturbing effects of the experiment.
Instead of viewing low-EE relatives as detached and neutral,
we realised that they were playing an actively supportive role.
We would never have made this important discovery if we had
tested all the patients in a laboratory away from their home
environment and their relatives. Indeed, Nick Tarrier did just
that as one of his experiments. In the laboratory the patients
from low-EE and high-EE homes produced skin conductance
records that were indistinguishable.

The impact of life events

What about life events? Could we also detect their impact on the patients? Since events were relatively uncommon, we could not look at each occasion of testing separately. For example, only four patients reported a life event before the first recording session. Therefore we pooled the data for all the three sessions for the seven patients who had experienced a life event before at least one of the sessions. In effect we were using patients as their own controls, comparing their responses on occasions preceded by an event with event-free sessions. From the beginning of the session the patients show a reduction in SF rate whether or not a life event has occurred. Once the relative enters the room the two graphs diverge. When an event precedes the recording, the patients respond to the relative with a steep rise in the SF rate which then remains high for the rest of the session. This shows that there is an interaction between the arousing effects of a life event and the presence of the relative, which neither on their own produces (Figure 4). Most of these seven patients lived with a high-EE relative, but the numbers are too small to separate out the recordings for the different types of relative.

Symptoms and stress

This experiment succeeded in establishing a link between two kinds of environmental stress that we knew could provoke attacks of schizophrenia, and a bodily response indicating a state of arousal of the nervous system. There is, however, a problem with using the concept of arousal since it is common to a number of different emotional states experienced by normal people, including pleasurable excitement as well as fear and anger. It also applies to the whole range of psychiatric conditions, including depression, which can take an agitated form. The challenge, then, was to show that the general state of high arousal was linked with specific symptoms of schizophrenia. We could not use delusions for this purpose since they are relatively long-term symptoms which do not fluctuate in intensity over minutes or even hours. What we

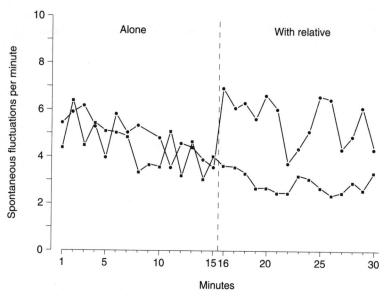

Figure 4 Mean number of spontaneous fluctuations per minute during the test period for seven patients on occasions preceded by a life event (circles) and the same patients on occasions when no life event had been experienced (squares). If a patient had two occasions succeeding a life event (or not), the mean of both was calculated. Patients who experienced (or did not experience) a life event on all three occasions are excluded from this graph

needed was an experience which came and went over a matter of minutes in order to look for associations with changes in the SF rate over the same period of time. The obvious choice was hearing voices, particularly as this is a common symptom in schizophrenia. The snag was how to determine when the patient was hearing voices. Of course we could simply ask the patient to tell us when this was occurring, but I had my doubts about relying on the patients to be accurate informants.

When I worked at Friern Hospital my research offices were adjacent to a house in the grounds in which lived twelve patients who were under my care. One of the men used to spend a lot of time sitting on the verandah, which was visible from my window. He often carried on a dialogue with invisible others, shouting and laughing at the top of his voice. Whenever I interviewed him to check on his progress I would ask him how much he was troubled by the voices. 'Voices, Doc?' he would query incredulously, 'I haven't heard voices for years.'

Charting 'voices'

As a result of several encounters of this kind I felt it was necessary to use a more objective and reliable indicator of auditory hallucinations. I had noticed that a number of patients who admitted to hearing voices showed characteristic eye movements. Their eyes would suddenly flick upwards and to one side, remain in that position for a few seconds, and then move back to a central position. If someone unexpectedly snapped their fingers next to one of your ears you would probably show the same response. With two colleagues, Ruth Cooklin and David Sturgeon,[35] I videotaped a few patients who showed these eye movements and we viewed the tapes independently. We found that we could agree most of the time on when the eye flicks began, although there was less consistency on when the eyes moved back to a central position again, presumably because the flick up and out was more abrupt than the shift back.

'Voices' and stress

We then set up an experiment in which a sample of patients who clearly showed these eye flicks had their skin conductance measured under two conditions: either sitting alone, or sitting with an experimenter who engaged them in conversation about neutral topics. We randomised the order of these two conditions so that some patients were alone first, while others started off sitting with the experimenter. The aim of introducing the experimenter was to see if the frequency of the voices would be reduced by interacting with a non-threatening person. We instructed the patients to raise their hand when they heard voices. The first thing we discovered in reviewing the videotapes was that the observers detected far more eye flicks than times when the patients raised their hand. Thus my reluctance to rely on the patients' reports was justified.

When we compared the time the patient was alone with the period spent talking to the experimenter we found that the number of eye flicks was significantly less during the sociable interaction. The importance of this observation is the practical advice that can be given to relatives and professional carers to attempt to engage the patient in conversation when they are obviously responding to auditory hallucinations. In order to test the hypothesis that had prompted the experiment, we superimposed the onset of eye flicks on the record of the SF rate. It was evident that most eye flicks coincided with an increasing SF rate. Thus we had established a link between a measure of arousal and one of the cardinal symptoms of schizophrenia. Unfortunately we were bedevilled by the ambiguity of the direction of cause and effect that we discussed in Chapter 3. We could not tell whether an increase in the patient's arousal triggered the voices or whether hearing the voices aroused the patient. And there our attempts to fill in the missing links in the chain of causality between environmental stress and episodes of schizophrenia have had to rest.

Visualising the brain in action

Since we halted our research into this difficult set of problems, the technology of functional brain imaging has developed. Unlike brain scans which produce a static picture of the structure of the brain, functional imaging generates information about the dynamics of the brain, allowing links to be made with transient phenomena like auditory hallucinations. Most methods of producing images of the functioning brain depend on the fact that when a region of the brain becomes more active the blood supply increases immediately to supply the brain cells with oxygen and glucose and to take away waste products. The technique used first to detect changes in the blood flow was to introduce a small amount of water tagged with radioactivity into the blood stream and to follow the pulse of radioactivity through the brain. More recently it was discovered that the magnetic properties of the hydrogen atoms in water distributed throughout the body and especially in the blood could be used to give more precise pictures of changes in blood flow. Functional magnetic resonance imaging (fMRI), as it is termed, is now the dominant technique in the imaging field.

Philip McGuire and his colleagues at the Institute of Psychiatry in London used a radioactive scanning technique in the early 1990s to measure blood flow through the brain in patients with schizophrenia. They chose patients who were hearing voices frequently and carried out a scan at this time and then repeated it five months later when the patients had improved as a result of treatment. This design uses patients as their own controls, comparing brain activity while hallucinating with that at a later time when the voices have faded or vanished. The main difference between the two sets of scans was that when the patients were hallucinating there was much more activity in the region of the brain on the left side that deals with the production of speech. In the vast majority of right-handed people the left side of the brain is concerned with speech, and nine of the twelve patients were right-handed. This result was a surprise since the expectation was that auditory hallucinations would be generated from the parts of the brain that deal with hearing and memory. The voices that patients hear are often those of familiar people repeating everyday phrases, so McGuire and colleagues expected that the region of the brain that stores what has been heard would be involved. The link with activity in the speech area, although not predicted by these researchers, fits with the observation that when words are accessed by a subject, blood flow increases to the front part of the brain and to the speech area. It also supports a theory proposed by several researchers that auditory hallucinations are actually a misinterpretation of the inner speech that continues in all of us just below the level of awareness. We can bring it into consciousness by making an effort to focus on it, a technique used by some writers such as James Joyce and known as tapping into the 'stream of consciousness'. Many children invent imaginary friends with whom they have conversations out loud, and some adults are aware of carrying on silent dialogues in their head when trying to make a decision. If auditory hallucinations and speech are indeed generated by the same region of the brain, there could be competition between them. This could explain the finding in our experiment that patients talking with another person showed less evidence of hearing voices than when they were alone.

These ideas were explored further by the group at the Institute of Psychiatry using the more recent technique of fMRI. They employed the same design of testing patients when they were hallucinating and then again three months later when they were much improved. This time they played a pre-recorded story to the patients while they were being scanned. This would be expected to activate the temporal lobe of the brain, the region which deals with memory for words. They found that the story produced less activity in the temporal lobe when the patients were hallucinating than when they had recovered. This result suggests that not only is there competition between auditory hallucinations and the patient's inner speech, but also with external speech produced by others. Many relatives complain that it is hard to get through to the patient at times, presumably because their attention is focused on the voices. Some patients learn to use a portable stereo recorder to compete with insistent voices and reduce their intensity, thus highlighting the practical value of such competition.

This work is promising but is still subject to the technical limitations of the measuring equipment: subjects have to remain lying down with their head inside a cylinder and fixed in place with a padded head restraint. The machinery is also quite noisy. Until the development of less cumbersome measuring techniques, the enormous advantage of recording the patient's responses to social situations of a known stress level will be beyond our reach.

| # The People versus the Professionals

Untreated illness

I have already pointed out ways in which the public view of psychiatric illness differs from the professional view. In this chapter the discrepancies will be explored in greater depth. One of the reasons for the different perspectives was formulated in Britain by David Goldberg, a psychiatrist, and Peter Huxley, a social worker, in 1980.[36] They described a series of filters which intervene between the distressed person in the community and the patient in a psychiatric ward. The first filter operates between the person who feels miserable or anxious, and the general practitioner. By no means all people who develop a depression or anxiety state seek help from their general practitioner. Some may not recognise that they are suffering from a treatable illness. Others, from past experience, may expect their doctor to show little sympathy. Yet others may wait for some weeks in the hope that their symptoms will resolve without treatment, and they may be proved right. It is only when surveys are carried out on the general population that untreated neurotic illness comes to light. In 1995 the Australian Health Department funded a national survey of mental health and wellbeing. A random sample of the whole adult population was selected and these participants were interviewed with a standardised schedule designed to generate psychiatric diagnoses. It emerged that four per cent of men and seven per cent of women had suffered from depression within the previous year, seven per cent of men and twelve per cent of women suffered from anxiety, and eleven per cent of men and five per cent of women abused substances, including alcohol. The striking finding was that sixty-two per cent of people with a diagnosed psychiatric disorder did not seek any professional help for their mental health problems. The proportion of such untreated illness varies from country to country and place to place according to the psychological sophistication of the public and the availability and accessibility of a primary care doctor or other medical help.

Body language

The next filter in the sequence is the general practitioner, who operates a selection process which is both intentional and unintentional. The intentional filter allows only one in twenty of the patients the general practitioner recognises as suffering from a neurotic illness to be referred to a psychiatric specialist. The general practitioner can manage the great majority of patients presenting with neuroses. Referral to the next level is usually because the patient has not responded to the first-line treatments prescribed, or that the illness is more severe or more complicated than usual, or that there is a serious risk of suicide. The unintentional filter results from the fact that most general practitioners fail to recognise the presence of a neurotic illness in about one in three patients. One of the reasons is inadequate training, and David Goldberg has spent much of his professional life devising and testing training programmes to correct this deficiency. Contributing to the difficulty of diagnosis is the fact that many patients present their distress as bodily symptoms. In the previous chapter I described the way the autonomic nervous system prepares the body for fight or flight in the face of a threat. These changes occur when a person becomes anxious even when there is no obvious danger. As we shall see, anxiety and depression are often inextricably mixed, so that these bodily

experiences are common to both states of mind. We can get
an idea of how large they loom in public consciousness by a
selection of phrases in common use: her heart sank, his skin
crawled, her legs turned to jelly, it brought a lump to my
throat, her heart was in her mouth, his head throbbed, it gave
me goosepimples, he went white with fear, I've got butterflies
in my stomach. Anxiety and depression are always accompanied by these bodily changes and the affected person may
focus on these rather than the psychological symptoms. This
creates a problem for the general practitioner who then has
to distinguish between the bodily response to psychological
distress and symptoms of physical disease. The general practitioner can sometimes feel impelled to embark on a prolonged and expensive series of laboratory investigations to
exclude a physical cause for the patient's complaints. There
is evidence that people in Western societies are becoming
increasingly aware of psychological experiences. Agony aunts
constantly give advice on how to deal with emotional problems, and television soaps captivate their viewers with the
emotions thrown up by fraught relationships. The growing
psychological sophistication of the public is not always
matched by the sensitivity of general practitioners, some of
whom have a blind spot for psychological problems and are
only interested in dealing with bodily complaints. Patients
learn to deal with this either by presenting their distress in
the form of physical symptoms or by seeking out a doctor in
the practice who is more responsive to psychological issues,
assuming that they have a choice.

Traditional healers

The situation in developing countries is very different. The
majority of the population are not psychologically minded
and there are few primary care physicians. This role is filled
by the traditional healer. Many traditional healers are rational
and resourceful people operating within a culture which ascri-

bes to them magical powers. But they are able to use their knowledge of the human condition to detect the emotional source of a problem even when, as is usual, it is presented as a physical complaint. Korean healers were described by Y. K. Harvey in 1976 as 'keenly intuitive and perceptive persons who make good use of their knowledge of people and human problems in helping their clients make the best of their situations. They give conservative advice, provide clients with outlets for potentially disruptive emotions, and get substantial help from the passage of time in solving clients' problems.'[37] No Western psychotherapist would feel slighted to be described in these terms.

There are a number of ways in which traditional healers are at an advantage compared with the general practitioner in the UK. They are usually much closer to their clients by virtue of living in a small community, and as a result know a great deal about the problematic relationships that exist. They also share the same world view as their clients, including beliefs about the causes and cures of diseases – which is not true of the general practitioner, whose medical explanation is almost always at variance with the popular views of causation. The traditional healer can assume that clients will understand the diagnosis and treatment without the necessity for long explanations. An account of a traditional healer in south India will illustrate these points. In the 1970s Mark Nichter studied Havik Brahmins in this region and found that women are expected to suppress the expression of emotion within the family.[38] They use bodily symptoms to signal distress, one in particular being known as *tale tirigutade*. This is translated as 'head turning' and is interpreted by most Western-trained doctors to mean giddiness or dizziness. However, traditional healers have another way of viewing the symptom. Nichter interviewed twenty-two clients of a traditional healer each of whom presented with this complaint. Among them were five individuals whose family was on the verge of breaking up, four people in economic crisis,

four women aged over twenty-five who were anxiously awaiting marriage, two people experiencing adjustment problems
following marriage, and one recently widowed woman who
had two daughters but no sons. The common theme is that
these problems induce uncertainty and disorientation, which
the individuals expressed in bodily terms as dizziness. The
healer would be very familiar with the family circumstances
of these clients and would be able to make the link between
these and the symptom with which they presented.

Mobilising social support

Whereas a Western psychotherapist would attempt to interpret the link between the patient's life circumstances and the
symptom, a healer would avoid this kind of approach. Family
relationships are not referred to explicitly in traditional societies, the subject being too sensitive; instead, the healer
explains the symptom in terms of shared beliefs about the
causes of illness, frequently within a spiritual context. For
instance, in Taiwan the healer's interpretation of the client's
complaints centres on a devil, a ghost or a god, which serves
as a symbol of a significant person in the client's life. Instead
of relationships with spouse, parents or neighbours being
spoken of directly, which would be unacceptable, a deceased
relative's spirit is identified as the source of the problem. In
this way, the real-life drama is depicted using the insub-
stantial world of the spirits. Having formulated a diagnosis
in acceptable terms, the healer will then prescribe a ritual
which often has the effect of strengthening the bonds between
the individual and the social group. For example, in Sri Lanka
the healer might recommend an exorcism ceremony which
involves a large group of participants, including musicians,
dancers, and people who represent the spirits, and which
continues from dusk till dawn. The cost of this production
would be well beyond the means of an individual or even a
single family, requiring cooperation between a large group of

relatives. Another strategy was used by an Indian healer studied by Nichter: he focused the attention of the family on the patient by involving family members in the preparation of time-consuming medicines and special meals. By these means the social resources around the patient are mobilised, emphasising the emotional support that is available.

The healer is called upon to activate the patient's social supports at times of stress, but many cultures use such resources routinely to help a bereaved person deal with loss. I explained in Chapter 1 how George Brown's research established a link between events representing loss and the development of depression. Is it possible that cultures that have retained methods of supporting the individual experiencing loss reduce the risk of depression? A review of such cultures will help us to answer this question. Each account represents the fieldwork of an anthropologist at a particular time and with a specific group of the people being studied. We should be cautious about assuming that they are true of an entire culture and that they are unchanging over time. Nevertheless they have important lessons to teach us about cultural resources on which bereaved individuals can draw.

Reciprocity in New Guinea

The Kaluli are a forest people of New Guinea whose society is based on the principle of reciprocity. If a thief steals a pig, the owner may steal a pig from the thief or demand money in compensation. The same concept is applied to losses in the non-material area of human relationships. The expected emotional response is anger, the intensity of which is in proportion to the loss experienced. Grieving is a response to devastating loss and represents an appeal for retaliation and compensation, just as if it were a possession that had been taken away unjustly. Grief is expressed publicly and worked through in weeping and song, not only at funerals but on many other occasions in ceremonies in which social support

is offered. Of course the loss of an intimate personal relationship cannot be compensated for in any meaningful way,
but the public display of anger and grief focuses the attention
of the group on the bereaved person and ensures that he or
she receives emotional support.

Grief in Iran

Iranian culture and history are dominated by the themes of
tragedy, injustice and martyrdom. These colour both classical
Persian poetry and modern novels, which are pervaded with
melancholy and despair. The culture places a high value on
sadness, which is regarded as an indication of personal depth.
Individuals growing up in the culture are taught to express
sadness appropriately and in a socially acceptable manner.
Most children first learn to grieve in the context of ceremonies for Iranian martyrs. So from an early age experiences
of loss, sadness and grief are assimilated into the suffering of
the wider community. In this way personal losses are placed
in the perspective of national tragedy, and bereaved individuals are never left alone with their grief. In Iranian culture
the emotional response to individual loss is incorporated in
the communal consciousness of historical tragedy.

Meditation in Sri Lanka

In 1985 the anthropologist Gananath Obeyesekere described
the coping style used by Sri Lankan Buddhists to deal with
loss.[39] In Buddhist philosophy, hopelessness lies in the nature
of the world and salvation is achieved by understanding and
overcoming that hopelessness. To do so one needs to recognise
the illusory nature of the world of sense, pleasure and domes-
ticity. A particular form of meditation is practised to diminish
the experience of loss. This is meditation on revulsion, the
purpose of which is to induce a sense of disgust for sensory
pleasure and to heighten awareness of the transitoriness of

the corporeal body. The body is imagined as 'a clay pot, polished on the outside, but full of faeces'. This image is applied to people close to the meditator, such as parents, spouse and children, and eventually extended to the whole of humankind. By these means a sense of loss may be coped with by weakening the emotional bonds to people in one's immediate social circle. Obeyesekere writes that it is almost impossible for a Sinhalese person to use words expressing sorrow without invoking Buddhist concepts: 'words used for personal emotional states resonate with the hopeless dilemma of mankind.'

We can see that Kaluli and Iranian culture both help people come to terms with loss by providing a network of social and emotional support around the individual which takes action at a time of crisis. The Sri Lankan Buddhist method of coping with loss is quite different in nature and much less compatible with Western ideologies. However, the importance of these examples is that each of the cultures has developed active resources which are available to the individual at a time of loss. How effective they are in preventing the development of depression is unknown. To discover this would require a series of longitudinal studies of people suffering a loss in different cultures. What is clear, however, is that in the absence of such resources in Western cultures it has become necessary to substitute natural support networks by professional inputs. George Brown's befriending scheme and our own couple therapy (see Chapter 4) are examples of professional substitution for the lack of supportive relationships.

The ritual of mourning

It was not always the case that Western societies lacked cultural procedures for dealing with loss. During the Victorian era and extending into the beginning of the twentieth century elaborate mourning rituals were observed. The clothes that the bereaved family should wear were specified, as was the length of a period of full mourning, to be followed by a time of half-mourning. European children observed the correct rituals in the same way as adults. Children mourned the death of a parent for twelve months, in the first six wearing the dull black and heavy crêpe of deepest mourning. For the next three months of ordinary mourning they wore black silk without crêpe, while in the final three months they were dressed in half-mourning colours. The bereaved wife was expected to wear 'widow's weeds', and straw was laid down outside the house to muffle the sounds of passing horses and carriages. Among observant Jews today the bereaved family is expected to remain in the home for seven days, during which time the men do not shave. The family is visited daily by relatives, friends and neighbours who bring them food, so that they do not have to get involved in household activities. The period of mourning ends after one year when a stone is erected over the grave.

The value of these rituals is that they specify how bereaved people should behave, and they mark them out as needing special treatment by their social circle. They also set a clear limit to the length of the mourning period and indicate when the bereaved person should cease to grieve and should re-enter life fully. The disappearance of these practices has left people at a loss to know how to behave; both the bereaved and their well-wishers. It has also posed a problem to the professionals: when does a normal bereavement response become a depressive illness? In the current WHO ICD-10 Classification of Mental and Behavioural Disorders there is a diagnostic category termed 'prolonged depressive reaction', which is meant to be used for bereavement reactions that last longer than six months, but this is clearly an arbitrary limit.

Shifts in diagnosis

Obeyesekere presents the challenging view that the use of the term 'depression' in the West is a medicalisation of the response to loss. In the absence of culturally prescribed coping strategies, it has become necessary to deal with the emotions consequent on a loss as though they were an illness and to treat the distress with medication. This concept is not applicable to manic-depressive illness, which has a strong basis in inheritance, but could be seen as relevant to the less severe forms of depression common in the general population. Once antidepressant medication was introduced, the pharmaceutical companies seized the opportunity to make large profits out of a very common 'condition' and pushed their products with massive advertising campaigns. These of course were targeted at psychiatrists and particularly at general practitioners, who treat ninety-five per cent of patients with neuroses, as noted by David Goldberg and Peter Huxley. One surprising effect of this propaganda was detected by Edward Hare,[40] a psychiatrist at the Maudsley Hospital. He reviewed the diagnosis of neurotic conditions recorded in the hospital for the period 1949–69, during which the first antidepressant drug was made available. He found that after its introduction there was a major shift away from the diagnosis of anxiety, which was replaced by the diagnosis of depression. How could this have happened?

There are four factors that contributed to this abrupt change in the way psychiatrists diagnose their patients. I have emphasised the first throughout this book, namely that there are no laboratory tests to back up a psychiatric diagnosis, so that the boundaries between conditions can waver back and forth, swayed by the climate of opinion and by the idiosyncratic beliefs of individual psychiatrists. The second is the understandable need psychiatrists have to feel that they can offer effective treatments. When a new treatment becomes available it tends to be prescribed for a wide range of conditions in the hope that they will respond. It takes some years for psychiatrists to narrow down the range of a new treatment to the patients for whom it really works. The advent of the first antidepressant medication opened up exciting possibilities for psychiatrists, who, given the flexibility of the system, opted for a diagnosis that they thought they could treat. The third factor is the competition between the pharmaceutical companies for a very lucrative market. It is in the interest of a company to sell a product on the basis that it has specific advantages over its competitors. An instructive example is provided by the introduction of the first antipsychotic drugs.

Selling a product

I have already described the introduction into psychiatry of the first antipsychotic drug, chlorpromazine (Largactil), in 1955. It rapidly cornered the market worldwide and in the first ten years more than thirty million prescriptions were issued. A few years after its debut, a pharmaceutical chemist, Paul Janssen, synthesised a new drug, haloperidol, which belongs to a different chemical family. It had similar effects on psychotic illnesses but was not obviously superior to chlorpromazine. Currently it costs $200 million to bring a new drug to the market, and these costs have to be recouped. The spin doctors in Janssen's company came up with the idea of marketing haloperidol as a specific treatment for mania, hoping to replace chlorpromazine for this condition. In fact haloperidol is less sedative than chlorpromazine and is consequently less useful for manic patients, who are often physically and mentally overactive and need to be calmed down. Nevertheless, so successful was the marketing campaign, that haloperidol is still linked with mania in the minds of psychiatrists decades later, long after the patent on haloperidol ran out.

Overlapping diagnoses

The fourth factor is the substantial overlap in symptoms between depression and anxiety. This phenomenon is well recognised by researchers who survey samples of patients with standardised interviews. Yet you would not learn this by consulting textbooks of psychiatry, which present anxiety and depression as distinct, well-demarcated conditions. The different views of anxiety and depression held by psychiatrists and by the patients suffering from them were highlighted by a study I conducted in 1978.[41] It involved twenty patients suffering from neuroses and ten experienced psychiatrists. They were each asked to rate feelings of depression and anxiety on eleven psychological and eleven bodily symptoms. For instance, they were asked to state whether when depressed their heart beat fast (bodily symptom) and if they wanted to die (psychological symptom). The patients were asked to rate their own unpleasant feelings, while the psychiatrists were asked to respond as they expected a typical neurotic patient would do. The ratings were then analysed to see how much overlap there was between the symptoms of anxiety and depression. A correlation of 1 would mean complete overlap. For the patients the correlation between the two lists of symptoms was 0.62, which indicates that a great many symptoms were common to both conditions. For the psychiatrists the correlation was zero: no overlap between depression and anxiety whatsoever. These senior and experienced psychiatrists maintained idealised concepts of depression and anxiety as crystallised conditions, which bore little relation to the experiences of their patients.

The reality was revealed two years before my study by a survey conducted by Phillip Snaith and his colleagues in Leeds.[42] They asked patients suffering from anxiety or depression to fill in two questionnaires, one relating to symptoms of anxiety, the other to symptoms of depression. Of the patients diagnosed by the clinicians as suffering from anxiety neurosis, only twenty-four per cent had scores that did not overlap with those of the depressed patients. Similarly, only twenty-six per cent of the patients diagnosed with depression had scores that were distinct from those of the anxious patients. Of the total group, seventy-three per cent fell into the middle range of scores and were considered by Snaith and his colleagues to represent 'anxiety-depressions'.

Given that the majority of patients with neuroses experience an equal balance of symptoms of anxiety and depression, it is easy for the clinician to focus on one or other cluster of symptoms and impose a diagnosis of 'pure' anxiety or 'pure' depression. This explains how the psychiatrists at the Maudsley Hospital were able to shift their diagnoses from anxiety to depression over a few years in response to the availability of antidepressants. You may be wondering how it was that these astute clinicians failed to notice that their patients who would have been given a diagnosis of anxiety previously did not improve on an antidepressant. The answer is that most antidepressant drugs have sedative effects and reduce the symptoms of anxiety as well as those of depression. To call them antidepressants is therefore understating the range of symptoms they may affect beneficially. So even some patients with predominant anxiety can respond well to antidepressants.

Genes and environment

A study of twins by Kenneth Kendler and his colleagues in 1987 throws an interesting light on the relationship between anxiety and depression.[43] They used the strategy of comparing single-egg (monozygotic) twins with two-egg (dizygotic) twins to attempt to sort out genetic from environmental influences (see Chapter 2). Single-egg twins have exactly the same genetic make-up, whereas two-egg twins have only half their genes in common, as with any pair of siblings. Any characteristic that is more commonly shared by the single-egg than by the two-egg twins is likely to be largely inherited, while characteristics that are equally shared by the two types of twin pairs are more likely to be environmental in origin. I need to stress that the environment is a very broad concept that stretches from complications at birth, through parental styles of upbringing, and viral infections, to toxins such as lead in the atmosphere. Kendler and his group used the Australian Twin Register to send questionnaires on depression and anxiety to nearly 3000 twin pairs of the same sex. From their analysis of the responses to the questionnaire, they concluded that what is inherited is a general liability to psychological distress and that the genes do not determine whether the individual will become depressed or anxious. It is the environment that shapes the general distress into a predominantly anxious or depressed form.

Loss and danger events

In 1980 George Brown and Robert Finlay-Jones,[43] an Australian psychiatrist, had carried out research on precisely this issue: the features of the environment that determine whether a person will develop anxiety or depression. I presented in Chapter 1 the work of Brown and Harris which established that the onset of depression was associated with events that represented a loss of something or some person valued by the depressed individual. Following this they moved on to enquire into the relationship between life events and the onset of anxiety. Brown and Finlay-Jones interviewed 164 women who were attending a general practice in central London. Using the Present State Examination (*see* Chapter 1) they identified those women who had sufficient psychiatric symptoms to pass the threshold for someone to need treatment. They classified them into predominant depression, predominant anxiety, and a mixture of the two: approximately one-third fell into each category. They focused on the women whose symptoms had started within the previous year and compared them with women who were psychiatrically healthy. They gave each woman the Life Events interview that Brown and Harris had developed for the research on depression, but added a further dimension to it. They had previously rated events by the severity of loss they represented, characterising losses as those of a person by death or separation, of the individual's physical health, of jobs, career opportunities, material possessions, or of a cherished idea, for example, the partner's fidelity. They extended the description of events to include those that threatened danger. They found that women with depression had experienced an excess of loss events in the three months before their symptoms began, replicating their previous results. Women with anxiety had experienced an excess of danger events, while those with mixed symptoms reported both more loss and more danger events than the healthy women. It appears from the findings of the genetic research by Kendler and the social research by Brown that it is the character of happenings in our environment that determines whether we become depressed or anxious, and not our constitution.

What the public want

I have argued with respect to neurotic illnesses that the public experience of depression and anxiety differs from the professional concepts of these conditions. The treatment preferred by the public is talking therapy, which is appropriate given the link, established by research, between the lack of a confiding relationship and the development of neuroses. The majority of psychiatrists and general practitioners view medication as the first line of treatment, whereas the public are suspicious of drugs and often do not take them even when they are prescribed. A series of three surveys of public attitudes in Great Britain were conducted between 1991 and 1997 under the auspices of the Royal College of Psychiatrists and the Royal College of General Practitioners. During the six years covered by the surveys, over ninety per cent of the respondents thought counselling should be offered to people suffering from depression, compared with less than a quarter recommending antidepressants. This type of drug was considered to be addictive by three-quarters of the people surveyed. A public education campaign run jointly by the two Colleges increased the proportion of people endorsing antidepressants by fifty per cent but did not change the view of their addictive nature.

Madness and violence

Turning to the psychoses, schizophrenia and manic-depressive illness, there also exists a wide discrepancy between the public and professional views of these disorders. The lay image of psychosis is epitomised in the phrase 'mad axeman'. The stereotype of the unpredictably violent psychotic person is constantly reinforced by the media, with headlines such as 'Schizophrenic raped three' and films such as *Psycho*. How close is this image to the truth? Some patients with psychosis commit violent acts and a small number kill others, but they represent a tiny proportion of all those with schizophrenia or manic-depressive illness. It is not a simple matter to determine whether people with psychosis are more or less violent than the general population. This is because violent acts tend to occur in the early phase of these illnesses, and to be committed by young men. In the general population it is also young men who are the most violent. So a comparison with the general population has to take account of age and sex. This form of analysis was carried out in 1998 by two professors of forensic psychiatry in London, Pamela Taylor and John Gunn.[45] They calculated that people with mental illness were no more likely than members of the general public to commit homicide. Furthermore, most murders by the mentally ill are of members of their own family. Random killing of strangers is very rare, although it is blazoned in banner headlines when it happens.

I led a team in a study of nearly 700 patients discharged from long-term care in two psychiatric hospitals. We followed up these patients five years after they had moved into homes in the community, most of them having staff on the premises to supervise the patients. We found that nine patients had committed assaults on members of the public. Some of these were serious, but fortunately nobody died. To put this in perspective, the violence that the public most fears was shown by just over one per cent of the patients over the course of five years. Given that violence by the mentally ill is in reality quite rare, how can we explain the prominent position it occupies in the mind of the public? It is not only uncontrolled violence that colours the stereotype of the mentally ill person but also unbridled sexuality. In every culture a central aim of the upbringing of children is the control of aggression and sexuality. These drives are very powerful and though they may be driven underground by the process of socialisation, they remain a disturbing subterranean force. A common way of dealing with unacceptable impulses is to deny them in oneself and to impute them to others, a psychological defence known technically as 'projection'. A tiny minority of people with psychosis show aggressive or sexually inappropriate behaviour, but that is enough for the public to tar all the mentally ill with the same brush. Once unacceptable feelings have been projected onto the mentally ill, they can be dealt with by ejecting from society the people tainted with them.

This process of expulsion dominated psychiatry in nineteenth-century Europe and America. Hundreds of asylums were constructed: in Britain alone over one hundred. The Victorians were very proud of their asylum building programme, which they saw as a public service. The asylums were typically sited outside towns and cities, far enough away not to be in the sight of the public, but not too remote to make the transport of patients difficult. One of the asylums my team studied, Friern Hospital, was built on a green-field site to the north of London, and the railway was extended to reach the hospital. The pride taken in these institutions is reflected in their ornamentation: Friern is an Italianate Gothic building with a frontage that is protected by the Department of the Environment. Its prestige is also evident from the fact that its foundation stone was laid by Prince Albert in 1851.

The rise and fall of the asylum

These institutions became little worlds in themselves, surrounded by high walls enclosing large grounds, often including a farm which produced vegetables and bred livestock for consumption by the staff and patients. With the help of the unpaid labour of the patients, some even produced a surplus which was sold to outside buyers. So successful in its own terms was the Victorian asylum that it was exported to all parts of the British Empire. After planting the Union Jack, almost the next step in colonisation was to build a lunatic asylum. The first public mental hospital in Greece was built on Corfu in 1838, four years after the British occupation of the Ionian Sea islands. I have visited various parts of Africa, India and the British West Indies and have frequently been confronted by buildings of an uncanny familiarity which housed psychiatric patients. The asylums the British built around the Empire were mainly for their own people: the natives had to rely on their own resources. As we shall see, their own resources proved superior to what the colonials had to offer.

Once the usefulness of the asylums was appreciated, all manner of people rejected by society were admitted, often for life. Some unmarried women who became pregnant were sent into asylums and never returned to their homes. As a result the number of inmates rapidly exceeded the capacity of the buildings and extensions were added. Even this did not suffice; and dense overcrowding occurred. Patients had to climb over other people's beds to reach their own. Friern Hospital was originally designed for 1000 patients but by 1952, one hundred years after its opening, its population had reached 2400. With overcrowding came squalor; the staff could not cope with the mass of patients, and physical abuse became common, eventually leading to public scandals. In Britain the number of psychiatric beds reached a peak in 1954 and then began to decline.

This turnaround was due to a number of factors, in addition to the public scandals. During the Second World War, army psychiatrists treated numerous young men who developed neuroses after facing terrible dangers and harrowing sights. Conditions that had been labelled 'shell shock' in the First World War under the mistaken belief that they were the result of concussion to the brain, were now diagnosed more appropriately as 'battle neurosis'. Removed from the front line to Netley Hospital in England and treated sympathetically, many of these psychiatric casualties made a full recovery. The psychiatrists experienced an antidote to the pessimistic views regarding recovery that pervaded the asylums. With the ending of the war, these young army psychiatrists moved into the asylums, bringing with them a fresh optimism and novel ideas about treatment, including group therapy which had been instituted in the army. A few years later in 1955, the first antipsychotic drug, chlorpromazine (Largactil), was introduced, making it possible to discharge patients who had seemed incurable. Psychiatry advanced behind the banner of community care and successive governments of both the left and the right endorsed the policy of eliminating the old asylums. By the year 2000, only fourteen of the 130 asylums in England and Wales remained open. A similar policy is being pursued in the rest of western Europe and in America, although in the USA the ferment which activated the asylum staff was not principally army psychiatrists, even though it did stem from the war. Conscientious objectors in the United States were obliged to do public service in psychiatric hospitals, and introduced into these institutions humanitarian attitudes which had not been eroded by the hospital regimen.

Outcome of schizophrenia around the world

Of course the revolution in psychiatric care never happened in the developing countries, because they had not invested in building asylums, and the colonial legacy was limited to a few such institutions in any one country. The great majority of people with schizophrenia and manic-depressive illness were cared for by their families as they had always been. Was this better for the patients than the professional care provided in the psychiatric institutions? From the 1970s onwards studies began appearing of the outcome of schizophrenia in developing countries. Prime examples are a study in Sri Lanka by Nancy Waxler,[46] an American researcher, and a study by Henry Murphy and Abdul Raman on the island of Mauritius off the coast of Africa.[47] This research suggested that people with schizophrenia actually suffered from fewer relapses of their illness in developing countries than in the West, despite the lack of availability of professional care, including anti-psychotic drugs for both treatment and maintenance. Before it could be taken seriously, this provocative result needed to be replicated in an international study using the same methods of assessment in all the countries being compared. This was achieved in the International Pilot Study of Schizo-phrenia, the WHO study described in Chapter 2. The samples of patients in the participating centres were followed up after two years and then five years in order to compare the course of their illnesses. At both time points patients with schizo-phrenia did conspicuously better in centres in developing countries, particularly Agra in India and Ibadan in Nigeria, than patients in Western centres.

There was a problem in interpreting this finding since the patients in this study were not representative of all the people with psychoses in the catchment area of the centre. This difficulty was a spur to the initiation of the successor WHO study, the Determinants of Outcome of Severe Mental Disorders (DOSMD), which was based on catchment area populations (*see* Chapter 2). Once again a two-year follow-up revealed a better outcome for patients in developing countries than for those in the West. Prompted by the intriguing finding of the first WHO study, in which I was involved, a psychologist, Elizabeth Kuipers, and I decided to use the DOSMD study to test a hypothesis about the possible cause of the differences in outcome. Since the expressed emotion of relatives was a powerful influence on the outcome of schizophrenia (*see* Chapter 3), could it be that relatives in developing countries were less likely to show high-EE attitudes?

There was already a suggestion that this might be the case from a study conducted in the 1980s by Marvin Karno and Janis Jenkins of Mexican-American families in Los Angeles.[48] One-third of the population of this west-coast city is made up of Mexicans, many of them illegal immigrants. They have largely retained their traditional style of life, with large extended families living together or nearby. Expressed emotion was measured in the relatives of patients with schizophrenia, and it emerged that the proportion who rated high, forty-one per cent, was considerably smaller than the equivalent figure of sixty-seven per cent for Anglo-American relatives in the same city.

Expressed emotion in Indian relatives

Encouraged by this result, we incorporated in the DOSMD project a substudy of relatives' EE in the centre in Chandigarh, north India. We selected Chandigarh because it encompassed two contrasting cultural environments, a city and a surrounding rural area, the characteristics of which are described in Chapter 2. Training in rating EE was given to two local fieldworkers, Harminder Bedi, an anthropologist, and Keerti Menon, a social worker. The training was conducted in English, but the interviews had to be given in one of the local languages, Punjabi or Hindi. Therefore the schedule was translated into these languages and then back-translated into English as a check on the accuracy of the translation. Following the standard procedure, relatives were interviewed at the time the patients made contact with the psychiatric services. The patients were then followed up one year later and the course of their schizophrenia charted.

The EE ratings of the urban relatives were analysed separately from those of the rural relatives, and the two sets of figures were compared with those for a sample of relatives in London. The Chandigarh city dwellers were much less critical than their counterparts in London, but surprisingly showed a similar amount of hostility. They rated very low on over-involvement, as did the rural relatives. The villagers expressed about half the amount of criticism compared with the urban relatives, and showed very little hostility. When these ratings were used to assign relatives to a high-EE category the differences between the three groups were striking: close to half of the London relatives were high-EE compared with thirty per cent of the Chandigarh urban relatives and only eight per cent of the villagers. This indicates a high level of tolerance by the rural relatives for the symptoms and behaviour associated with schizophrenia. Relatives living in the city of Chandigarh are about midway between the villagers and the London relatives for high-EE, suggesting that education and an urban lifestyle diminish tolerance for people with schizophrenia.

We compared the relapse rate for the Chandigarh patients with a group of patients with schizophrenia making first contact with the psychiatric services in London. The Indian patients had half the relapse rate of the London patients and their better outcome was largely accounted for by the low level of EE of their relatives. It seems that our hunch was right: the support relatives are able to give the patients is a major factor in producing a better outcome for schizophrenia in developing countries. Of course these results raise another question: what is it about life in rural settings that enables carers to maintain low-EE attitudes to the patients? To date no research has been directed at answering this question, but there are some educated guesses which are worth presenting.

Influences on EE

In traditional societies the causes of any illness are usually believed to lie outside the control of the patient. Illness is often ascribed to angered spirits, black magic worked by envious people against the patient, or simply fate. This type of explanation absolves the patient from any responsibility for falling ill. In contrast, in the West patients are increasingly held responsible for their illnesses. Patients with heart or lung disease are told they have brought it on themselves by choosing an unhealthy lifestyle. Mentally ill people are exhorted to 'pull yourself together'. Relatives become critical when they think the patients are in control of their actions and could behave properly if they really wanted to.

Another influential factor may be the extended family, in which a large number of relatives share the burden of caring for the patient. Hence no one individual is greatly stressed by the demands of being a carer. It is not uncommon in Western cities to find a middle-aged patient with long-standing schizophrenia being cared for by a single relative, often an elderly mother. It is hardly surprising that high levels of negative emotions develop in this situation. A further advantage of the extended family is the choice of relationships it offers the patient. If one relative has high-EE attitudes there are plenty of others with whom the patient can choose to spend time. Traditional families are also contrasted with the typical

Western nuclear family in restricting the expression of conflict within the family circle. Such families have ways of dealing with disagreements which avoid blow-ups and open dissension. They are probably aided in this by the acceptance of a hierarchy of authority based on seniority and gender, which has been eroded in the West.

While staying with a Muslim extended family in India I observed behaviour that puzzled me. The group of thirty-five people consisted of five brothers and their families living in a three-storey house. The women lived on the upper floors and never ventured into the rooms on the ground floor. I found that when one of the brothers was offered a cigarette, sometimes it was accepted and sometimes refused. I also noticed that the oldest brother would never give a command directly to one of the young boys, but would use one of the other brothers as an intermediary. I waited until I was alone with the most Westernised of the brothers and expressed my puzzlement to him. He seemed surprised that I was unaware of the convention that a man was not allowed to smoke in the presence of a senior male. The chain of command I had observed was a result of the rule that the senior male should not communicate directly with the most junior members of the hierarchy.

Finally, the nature of the work environment may play a part. In agrarian economies in developing countries there are still many unspecialised jobs available, such as minding the livestock, which do not demand a high level of skill. Thus even quite disabled people can do a useful job and feel that they are contributing to the family economy, since many enterprises are cooperatives run by the extended family. Furthermore there is not the insistence on time-keeping and productivity which are increasingly dominating the workplace in the West. It is obviously easier for a family to accept a member with schizophrenia who does something useful, however low-key, than one who sits around the home all day totally unoccupied.

Whatever the factors contributing to the development of high-EE attitudes may turn out to be, the evidence is strong that the urban environment in the West is inimical to people who have developed a schizophrenic illness. Could it also play a role in bringing it on in the first place? That question is addressed in the next chapter.

| # Do Cities Drive Us Mad?

The ecology of cities

The transition from hunter-gatherer to cultivator of the land anchored human communities in particular locations. As trade between communities flourished and central political control was established, villages grew into towns and towns into cities. Cities act as attractors to migrants from the countryside and inexorably increase in size. This process is still occurring: Mexico City is now one of the largest conurbations in the world, with 20 million inhabitants. While rural migrants in developing countries tend to build shanty towns from scrap materials on the periphery of cities, the pattern of settlement and growth is quite different in developed countries. One of the first descriptions of this process was written by Richard Faris and H. Warren Dunham in 1939 in relation to Chicago.[49] They saw the city as consisting of a series of concentric rings, each of which they called a zone. The central zone is dominated by businesses and places of entertainment, and few people live there. Western cities tend to expand from the centre outwards into the next zone, which is therefore known as the zone in transition. Since it is more profitable to build offices and shops than houses, domestic housing in the zone in transition is allowed to deteriorate structurally prior to its demolition. The rents are low, and affordable by the poorest sections of society. The surrounding zones increase in affluence as one moves further from the zone in transition, with a progressively greater proportion of owner-

occupiers until one reaches the outer zones constituting suburbia, where most people own their own homes. Most
Western cities fit into this pattern, although there are local
variations. For example, in London the many open spaces
are seen as desirable places to live near, which disrupts the
concentric zoning somewhat. Furthermore, after the Second
World War a Labour government restricted the expansion of
office building in the centre. This removed the threat hanging
over the zone in transition, which began to be recolonised by
the middle classes, who were becoming fed up with increasingly tedious commuting. This process, known as gen-
trification, only made sporadic inroads into the zone in
transition, which still retains much of its economically depressed character. As a consequence of the low rents, the zone in
transition is the first part of the city in which new immigrants
settle. Once they become economically well established, the
immigrants tend to move out to more salubrious zones. Thus
the Jews first settled in the East End of London in the sixteenth
century when Oliver Cromwell allowed them back into
England and later moved peripherally towards the northern
suburbs. Over time the East End has lost its Jewish character
as these immigrants were replaced by a wave of Bangladeshis
during the 1960s and '70s.

Distribution of illness in cities

Faris and Dunham studied the cases of schizophrenia and
manic-depressive psychosis admitted for the first time to
a central clinic in Chicago and to the state hospitals, and
calculated the incidence rates (*see* Chapter 2) for the different
districts. They found that the incidence of schizophrenia was
highest in the central zone and fell off peripherally in every
direction. They also looked specifically at the largest ethnic
minority group, the African-Americans. The rate for African-
Americans living among their own group was low, but those
living in predominantly white areas had a significantly higher

rate. As always with a cross-sectional study, these findings can be interpreted in two opposing ways. It is possible that the poor socio-economic conditions in inner-city areas produce a high rate of schizophrenia (the social breeder hypothesis). Alternatively, people predisposed to the illness may drift into the central zones of the city before the first appearance of the illness (the social drift hypothesis). Using similar arguments, African-Americans with little social support from their peers may be more likely to develop schizophrenia, or those with a susceptibility for the illness may shun their mates and seek isolation from their own group. I will return to these possibilities when considering African-Caribbean populations in the UK. In contrast with schizophrenia, admissions for manic-depressive psychosis were randomly scattered over the city, with no concentration in the central zones. Edward Hare,[50] a British psychiatrist, took the research a step further by studying the city of Bristol in 1955 and examining three main characteristics of the different districts, defined as electoral wards. He was interested in the proportion of single-person households (an index of social isolation), the mean rateable value (a measure of economic status) and the population density (relating to overcrowding). As in Faris and Dunham's study, the wards with the highest incidence of schizophrenia were all clustered together in the city centre, whereas other diagnostic groups, such as manic-depressive psychosis, neurosis and senile dementia, were distributed randomly throughout Bristol. The high rates of schizophrenia were not linked with economic status nor with overcrowding, but with the proportion of single-person households. This enabled Hare to formulate the opposing hypotheses more precisely: either social isolation predisposes to schizophrenia, or 'segregation' takes place and emotionally isolated people move into the lodging-house areas.

Social drift and social causation

Controversy over the interpretation of these results continued for some decades, but then died down when two further studies, one British, the other American, seemed to provide a conclusive answer. The British study was conducted in the 1960s by Tilda Goldberg and S. Morrison and concerned not geographical drift but social drift.[51] Not only is schizophrenia concentrated in the poorest locations in cities, but patients presenting with the illness for the first time are over-represented in the lowest social classes. Goldberg and Morrison argued that if this is due to a causative influence of low social class, then the patients' fathers should also show the same distribution. They focused on fathers rather than mothers since many women work in the home, which is hard to classify economically. Their approach was quite sophisticated: they argued that since people tend to improve their economic condition during their working life, it would be unfair to compare the patients at the beginning of their careers, when schizophrenia tends to first appear, with their fathers at the same point in time, when they would have been working for twenty years or more. A fairer comparison would be with their father's occupation at the time of the patient's birth, when the age of the father would be comparable with that of the patient on falling ill. This information was simple to obtain since father's occupation is recorded on all birth certificates. They found as expected that the patients showed the usual bulge in the lowest occupational classes at the time they fell ill. However, the social class distribution of their fathers did not differ from that of the general population. Their conclusion was that the patients drifted down the social scale from their fathers' position before the illness developed.

There is some support for this notion from anecdotal accounts of the school histories of people who go on to develop schizophrenia. Generally they keep up with their peers academically until adolescence. Then they often fail to fulfil

their earlier promise and leave school with few if any qualifications. Of course adolescence is a turbulent time for most
children, and many experience disruption to their studies
without it having any long-term effect on their careers. But
those with a predisposition to schizophrenia find it an uphill
struggle to make up for their lack of higher education and are
often forced into unskilled jobs. Thus they may not match up
to their family's level of social standing. Not all histories are
so dismal: some people manage to complete a university
degree before they fall ill. In general the earlier the illness
strikes, the more devastating is its effect on the person's
educational career and social development.

Mobility in Detroit

Twenty years after generating the original controversy,
Dunham returned to the problem.[52] This time he studied the
city of Detroit, an American centre of the car industry. He
identified two contrasting districts, one affluent – Connor-
Burbank – and the other working class – Cass. He monitored
all admissions for schizophrenia from these two districts over
a period of time, and found that the rate in Cass was three
times that in Connor-Burbank. He then divided the patients
into those who had lived in the district for more than five
years, and those who had moved into the district within the
past five years. The excess rate in Cass was almost entirely
due to the mobile patients. When these were excluded from
both groups the two rates became almost identical. Thus
Dunham felt he had shown that the high rate in impoverished
city areas is due to people moving in prior to the development
of a schizophrenic illness. When he looked at the places the
mobile patients had come from, they were not other parts of
Detroit but small towns outside the city.

   The Goldberg and Morrison study provided evidence that
poor socio-economic conditions do not directly contribute to
the causation of schizophrenia. Indeed if they did, one would

expect to see major variations in the incidence of schizophrenia with economic booms and busts, but the incidence
has been remarkably steady regardless of major international
upheavals such as the Great Depression and the two World
Wars. Hare demonstrated that the distribution of schizophrenia was linked with single-person households, and Dunham's second study suggested that people predisposed to
schizophrenia drifted into areas of the city where they could
find anonymity. And there the matter rested for over thirty
years, with a general feeling of satisfaction that the argument
had been settled.

Mobility in Nottingham

Then several papers were published which raised the dust.
One reported a small-scale study with a similar design to
Dunham's second survey in Detroit. This was carried out in
the British city of Nottingham, one of the centres taking part
in the WHO DOSMD study described in Chapter 2. Glynn
Harrison and his team collected sixty-seven patients with
schizophrenia presenting for the first time to the psychiatric
services during the two years 1978–80.[53] They charted the
areas of social deprivation in Nottingham and found as
expected that most of them were clustered in the centre of
the city, although there were scattered pockets of deprivation
in suburban zones. The incidence rate for schizophrenia in
the most deprived area was three times that in the most
affluent area, closely echoing Dunham's finding. High rates
were also found in the deprived areas situated in suburbia.
Harrison and his colleagues examined the mobility of the
patients in the five years before their first contact with the
services, just as Dunham had done. But here the similarities
between the two studies ended. Only eleven of the Nottingham patients had moved into the city in the preceding
five years, and they had settled randomly throughout the
various zones and did not account for the concentration of

cases in the deprived areas. Harrison's group took the argument one step further by looking at the place of birth of their patients. They found that a great excess of patients were born in areas of social deprivation. The Nottingham results directly contradict those from Detroit and suggest that social drift does not account for the link between social deprivation and high rates of schizophrenia. Could the discrepancy between the findings be due to the time lag of twenty years between the data collection in the two sites, or to different social conditions on either side of the Atlantic? We can only speculate about these possibilities, but fortunately the controversy has been overtaken by two large-scale studies which have employed a powerful method.

Linking records

There is a long tradition in northern European countries of keeping records on all their citizens. In Scandinavia it has been the responsibility of the parish priest for several hundred years to record significant events in the lives of his parishioners. These parish records are invaluable historical documents, chronicling changes in lifestyle over the centuries. National registers developed out of this tradition and because they cover the whole population, yield extremely useful data for research. Unfortunately national registers are also open to political exploitation, and the murder by the Nazis of over 100,000 mentally ill people naturally sensitised people to their dangers. So strong was public opposition in Germany that their national register was closed down some years ago, and this has been the fate of other European registers. The two studies that represent the greatest challenge to the social drift theory made use of national registers.

Swedish conscripts

In 1992 two British psychiatrists, Glyn Lewis and Anthony David, teamed up with two Swedish psychiatrists, Sven Andreasson and Peter Allebeck, to utilise data from a survey and a national register maintained in Sweden.[54] National service is still obligatory for Swedish men, and during 1969–70 a survey was conducted on all 50,456 young men called up for national service. The survey captured ninety-five per cent of the male population of Sweden in the age group eighteen to nineteen years. Among other questions, they were asked where they lived when they were growing up. Their place of upbringing was assigned to one of the following groups: the three biggest cities in Sweden, towns with more than 50,000 inhabitants, towns with fewer than 50,000 inhabitants, and the country. The data from the conscript survey were linked with the National Register of Psychiatric Care, which recorded admissions to psychiatric hospitals. This register was closed in 1983 so that it was possible to follow up the conscripts for fourteen years (1969–83) and identify those who were admitted for the first time with a diagnosis of schizophrenia. The highest incidence of schizophrenia was in the men brought up in one of the three cities (51.4 per 100,000), and was progressively lower for large towns, small towns, and the country, for which the rate was 31.2 per 100,000. This finding eliminates drift in the few years before the emergence of schizophrenia as an explanation for the concentration in cities. But the conscript survey did not ask where the men were born. The next study to exploit national registers did address this question.

Dutch registers

A study by Machteld Marcelis and his colleagues used two kinds of national register maintained in the Netherlands, which has experienced a great increase in urbanisation since the Second World War and is today one of the most densely populated countries in Europe. The Dutch Central Bureau for Statistics records all live births by sex. The Dutch National Psychiatric Case Register, like its equivalent in Sweden, records all admissions to psychiatric hospitals. First psychiatric admissions for psychosis between the years 1970 and 1992 were obtained from the Case Register and the place of birth of these patients was traced through the records of the Central Bureau for Statistics. Marcelis and his group found that people born in the most densely populated areas had the highest incidence of psychosis.[55] The strongest link with urban birth was found when they restricted the patients to those with narrowly defined schizophrenia. Applying this diagnosis, the incidence was twice as high for those born in the most urban areas as for those born in the least densely populated areas. These two studies have used the most sophisticated scientific methods available and have strongly supported the proposition that being born and brought up in cities increases the risk of developing schizophrenia in adult life. They have not been able to identify those aspects of city life that drive people crazy but they have provided a strong impetus for others to investigate this question. In the next chapter I will present the mental health problems of ethnic minority groups in the UK and discover what light they throw on the dangers of living in a city.

| # A Black and White Issue

Immigration to the UK

Since the Second World War Britain has increasingly become a multicultural society. The influx of peoples from all parts of the globe has brought to the attention of psychiatrists the fact that some immigrant groups appear to be more prone to severe mental illnesses than others. This awareness has raised sensitive political issues, as well as reviving fears that cities may be mentally unhealthy places. The particular group around which the political storm has raged are the African-Caribbean immigrants. At the end of the Second World War there was a desperate shortage of labour affecting the infrastructure of the country, mainly transport and the health service, which was nationalised in 1948. Vigorous recruiting campaigns were held in the West Indies to attract men to work as bus and train drivers and conductors, and women as nurses. These were successful and shiploads of West Indians came to the UK during the next ten years until the Immigration Acts of the early 1960s halted the flow. During the same period there was a massive influx of people from the Indian subcontinent following partition and independence in 1947. As a form of shorthand I shall use the term 'Asian' to refer to people from the Indian subcontinent, while recognising that it includes groups with widely differing languages, religions and cultures. Similarly the term 'African-Caribbean' encompasses people from islands with different dominant languages, religions and histories, and – in the case of Trinidad – distinct ethnic groups.

Like the African-Caribbean population, the Asian migrants were attracted by the lure of economic betterment, but no recruiting campaigns were held in India or Pakistan. In London both groups settled in the zone in transition, but in different parts of it. The African-Caribbeans were concentrated in Brixton and Notting Hill Gate, while the Asians chose Southall and the East End, from which the Jewish community had already begun to relocate to the more affluent outer zones. Unlike India, which has succeeded in absorbing successive waves of conquerors, the British West Indies were strongly oriented towards the UK and British culture, albeit a version that existed in an Edwardian time warp. Most respectable African-Caribbean homes both in the West Indies and the UK maintain a front parlour, in which the best china is displayed in a cabinet and which is reserved for entertaining guests. Britain was viewed as the mother country and the expectation was of being welcomed by the British, particularly as many of the immigrants were recruited to leave their homes and settle in the UK. The shock of meeting almost uniformly racist attitudes ('NO COLOUREDS, NO INDIANS, NO DOGS') was therefore much greater for the African-Caribbean immigrants than for the Asians, who may never have expected to be treated as anything other than aliens.

Rates of mental illness among African-Caribbeans

From the 1960s onwards studies have been appearing regularly in the psychiatric press purporting to show that African-Caribbean people have a much higher incidence of schizophrenia than the white population. Alongside these alarming publications have been reports that African-Caribbeans are more likely to be admitted to psychiatric units against their will than whites, that they are over-represented among the population of forensic psychiatric units, and that they receive higher doses of medication and are less likely to be offered psychotherapy than the whites. It is hardly surprising that the black community has responded with accusations of racism against white psychiatrists acting in concert with the police, who become involved in compulsory admissions, and the criminal justice system, which commits patients to forensic psychiatric institutions. There is an added force and bitterness to these protestations, given the findings of several official enquiries of widespread racism in the British police force, manifested as tardiness and ineptitude in investigations of a number of blatantly racist murders of young black people.

Psychiatry and social control

The precedent of the Soviet abuse of psychiatry, discussed in Chapter 2, has been cited as evidence that mentally healthy people have been deliberately misdiagnosed as suffering from schizophrenia with the aim of exerting social control over dissident members of society. White British psychiatrists have been portrayed as 'thought police' stifling the legitimate protests of black people against an unjust and racist society. These political accusations were fuelled by a book published in 1982 by two British psychiatrists, Roland Littlewood and Maurice Lipsedge.[56] Littlewood trained both as an anthropologist and a psychiatrist. They studied a series of African-Caribbean patients with a diagnosis of schizophrenia and drew attention to the high proportion who expressed delusions of a religious nature. They considered that some of the religious beliefs were within the range of accepted ideas of the evangelical churches to which the patients belonged and hence should not have been identified as delusions. This issue has been extensively aired in Chapter 2 in the discussion on the nature of delusions. Littlewood and Lipsedge also noted that twice as many African-Caribbean patients had their diagnosis changed in the course of their contact with services than white patients. They suggested that either British doctors found it hard to come to a conclusion about their diagnosis, or that the patients did not fit easily into the standard pigeonholes. The message that politically minded people took from this book was that black people who were essentially in good mental health were being wrongly diagnosed as having schizophrenia.

Because of the absence of any objective tests to validate psychiatric diagnosis, the accusation of misdiagnosis is very difficult to counter. In 1998 an attempt was made to investigate this issue at the Maudsley Hospital in London. Robin Murray, professor of psychiatry there, brought over a black psychiatrist from Jamaica, Fred Hickling, who was himself politically active in the controversy.[57] Therefore if he had any bias, it would be to prove that white psychiatrists were making diagnostic errors on black patients. He interviewed a series of patients of the Maudsley Hospital using a standardised clinical examination, the Present State Examination (PSE). He made his own diagnoses in ignorance of the diagnoses made by the local white psychiatrists. The two sets of diagnoses were then compared. There were major discrepancies between the two lists, but these were not linked to the ethnicity of the patients. Disagreements between the Jamaican psychiatrist and the British psychiatrists were just as common for white patients as for black patients. These exemplify the well-known mismatch between research diagnoses and the diagnoses made by clinical psychiatrists, but do not reveal any ethnic bias. This one study will not put the controversy to rest since racism undoubtedly exists in psychiatry as in other British institutions, and the charge of misdiagnosis is difficult to counter. However, it obscures a question of crucial importance: if this difference in incidence rates is real, what does it tell us about the nature of schizophrenia? Epidemiologists the world over become very excited when they find that the incidence of a disease is significantly higher in one human group than in another, because one can then look for other differences between the groups that might give clues to the cause of the disease, just as John Snow did by mapping the cases of cholera in London.

Psychosis in the West Indies

Together with my colleagues, Rosemarie Mallett, a sociologist, and Dinesh Bhugra, a psychiatrist,[58] I wished to investigate one obvious possibility, namely that the incidence of schizophrenia was high in the West Indies, and that the immigrants to the UK were simply reflecting the susceptibility of the populations from which they had come. To answer this question we would need to mount a study of the incidence of schizophrenia in a Caribbean island, a venture that had never been attempted before. A small island is an ideal location for an epidemiological study as the population is contained within clear boundaries and it is feasible to cover a large section of it with a survey. We chose the island of Trinidad since there was a reasonable number of psychiatrists working there, we had already established good relationships with some of the key figures, and several of the psychiatrists were keen to be involved with the research. All the psychiatrists who took part were black Trinidadians, so the question of a racist bias in diagnosis should not intrude. Furthermore, at the start of the study in the early 1990s, Dinesh Bhugra trained all the participating psychiatrists to use the PSE. When wind of this study reached the UK during the planning stage, a group of psychiatric activists wrote to me expressing their disquiet at what they saw as a racist attempt to prove that black people were more likely to go mad than white people. I felt that by attempting to block our study the activists were spoiling their own case, as they were removing the impetus to investigate another possibility, that life in Britain including the experience of racial harassment, might be driving black people mad. Therefore I ignored their warnings and went ahead with the Trinidad study.

The result was clear-cut: the incidence of schizophrenia in Trinidad was no higher than among whites in the UK. This finding was confirmed in 1999 by a second study carried out in collaboration with us by George Mahy on the island of Barbados,[59] the home of Rosemarie Mallett, and a third study on Jamaica conducted in 1993 by Fred Hickling and Pamela Rodgers-Johnson.[60] Thus we could discount the explanation that black people were particularly susceptible to schizophrenia. But there were still several other theories that needed to be examined. One rather subtle idea is that of selective migration, which also capitalises on the inherited basis of psychosis. This postulates that people carrying the genes for schizophrenia are less attached to their family and friends and therefore more likely to migrate than those who do not share the genes. Thus if you were able to compare the migrants with the stay-at-homes, the former group of people would contain more of the genes for schizophrenia than the latter. The main problem with this theory is that it cannot be tested at present since we do not have biological markers for genes that may predispose to schizophrenia. There are other objections to this theory: since African-Caribbean people living in the UK also have a higher incidence of manic-depressive illness, one would have to postulate that the genes for manic-depressive illness also impel people to migrate. Furthermore, the process of selective migration cannot be specific to one group of people but must operate for all migrants who are making a free decision to leave their country of origin, as opposed to those who are forced to leave by racial or political persecution. If this is so, then it is crucial to study the incidence of schizophrenia in other migrant groups who chose to come to the UK. The obvious group for comparison is the Asian population, and that is why my colleagues and I included them in our study of the incidence of schizophrenia.

Asians and African-Caribbeans in London

As already noted, the main migration from India occurred over the same period as that from the West Indies and for the same reason of economic betterment. The Asian migrants also faced racial prejudice and harassment, but had no expectation of being integrated into the 'mother country'. If selective migration were operating one would expect the Asians to have as high an incidence of schizophrenia as the African-Caribbeans. In order to collect enough patients to make reliable calculations we needed to focus on areas of London containing large numbers of the groups in question. The region of south-east London around the Maudsley Hospital has a high proportion of African-Caribbean residents – as much as twenty per cent in some districts – but very few Asians. On the other hand, Southall has a large Asian population. Therefore we selected these two areas for our study, and collected all new cases of schizophrenia making contact with the psychiatric services over the two-year period 1991–3. The national census took place during our study and for the first time asked people to indicate which ethnic group they felt they belonged to. This was of great value to us in determining the sizes of the ethnic minority populations to calculate the incidence rates. Previously these had been estimated indirectly from other sources of information and could have been far from accurate.

Hopes and achievements

Our aim was more ambitious than simply comparing incidence rates between white, African-Caribbean and Asian groups, important though that was. We were also concerned to identify possible aspects of life in Britain for an ethnic minority group that might be stressful enough to provoke schizophrenia. We needed a measure of racial harassment, and Dinesh Bhugra developed one from the life events interview of

George Brown and Tirril Harris. Called the Racial Life Events Schedule, Bhugra translated it (and other instruments to be used) into the Asian languages current among the population of Southall. We also developed two other measures, one being an assessment of the gap between expectations and achievement on the basis of the following argument. The African-Caribbean immigrants were lured to the UK with the promise of good jobs, but their children have not done well. The boys in particular have failed to advance academically and have a high rate of unemployment. It was the second generation who were entering the period of risk for schizophrenia at the time of our study, and who might be expected to be bitterly disappointed by their poor prospects compared with the high hopes with which their parents arrived in the UK and which they presumably transmitted to their children. We built on an existing instrument created by Parker and Kleiner in the United States for a study of black Americans in the 1960s. Curiously this pioneering work had never been followed up. We covered five domains of life: academic achievement, employment, housing, finance, and social standing.

Who do you think you are?

The other area we wished to investigate was cultural identity. We considered that the African-Caribbean settlers in the UK aspired to be accepted by the white majority and that many would move away from their traditional lifestyle in the hope of becoming assimilated, but that this was doomed by the rejecting attitudes of the whites. Hence they would find themselves in the stressful situation of being between two cultures, to neither of which they fully belonged. In contrast, we postulated that the Asians would have less desire for assimilation and would prefer to remain immersed in their traditional way of life. We obviously needed a measure of cultural identity and we constructed one each for the Asian and the African-Caribbean groups with the help of anthropologists. When we

compared the two versions we found that there was considerable overlap and we were able to amalgamate them into
one schedule with minor variations for each ethnic group.
The items included covered such issues as preferred foods,
mode of dress, language, reading matter, television programmes and films, and admired figures in public life.

The design of the study needs some explanation. If we
simply compared the patients from the three ethnic groups
we would not know whether any differences between them
were attributable to their ethnic backgrounds or to the different rates of schizophrenia. Therefore we needed control
groups of healthy people from the same ethnic groups as the
patients. This is known as a case–control study and is a
standard epidemiological design for identifying risk factors
for diseases. We carried out random door-knocking to collect
healthy controls for the patients and interviewed them with
the same collection of schedules.

Ethnic minorities in The Netherlands

The first step in analysis was to calculate the incidence rates,
since if there was no difference between them, there would
be nothing to explain. In fact the rate of schizophrenia for
African-Caribbean participants was double that for whites,[61]
confirming the results of many previous studies. The rate
for Asians was slightly higher than that for whites, but the
difference could easily have occurred by chance. Therefore
the explanation of the high rate in African-Caribbeans in
terms of selective migration was most unlikely, since it did
not apply to the Asians. Just after the end of our study, in
1994, a paper was published by two Dutch researchers, Jean-
Paul Selten and Arno Sjiben.[62] They had studied the incidence
rates of schizophrenia among various immigrant groups in
The Netherlands and compared them with the rate for the
white Dutch population. They found high rates among Caribbean immigrants from Surinam and the Dutch Antilles, in

harmony with our results, but also among immigrants from Morocco. However, immigrant Turks did not have a high rate. These interesting results suggest that there are particular experiences, provoking the development of schizophrenia, which affect some ethnic minority groups but not others. They underline the importance of our comparisons between African-Caribbeans and Asians in the UK.

Social disadvantage

Our attempt to obtain information on racial harassment from the ethnic minority subjects was a failure. Very few respondents were able to report verifiable incidents that could be included as racial life events. Either such occurrences are actually rather rare or people were reluctant to reveal them to the interviewers at the time of our survey. The recent public enquiries into racism in the police force may have increased people's willingness to speak on such issues. Even if racist events are infrequent in any individual's experience, a single racist murder, such as that of Stephen Lawrence in London, can terrorise a community for years to come. We decided that it would be more important in future studies to assess the subjects' perception of the climate of racism, rather than restricting ourselves to objective evidence.

To our surprise, the enquiry into expectations and achievements yielded few significant findings. The unemployment rate was certainly appallingly high among the patients: about half the white and Asian patients were without a job at first contact with the psychiatric services, as were eighty-five per cent of the African-Caribbean patients. However, for each ethnic group the unemployment rate among the patients was about double that of the healthy controls. It is impossible to tell from this cross-sectional picture whether the personal difficulties leading up to the appearance of schizophrenia were responsible for the lack of a job, or whether unemployment contributes to the development of schizophrenia. What we found difficult to account for was that, despite the tiny minority of African-Caribbean patients in work, the patients did not depict a large gap between their expectations of employment and their achievements in the job market. Perhaps they had already adjusted their expectations to the reality of an unemployment situation which had existed for some decades. The only area in which the African-Caribbean patients differed from their controls was that of housing. The patients felt that their current housing situation was considerably worse than they had expected it to be, whereas this did not apply to their controls. We found that African-Caribbean patients were more likely to be living in council accommodation than white or Asian patients, but we did not collect information on the quality of housing so cannot corroborate the patients' perception. Could poor housing conditions contribute to schizophrenia? It would certainly explain the concentration of schizophrenia in the zone in transition, but the evidence for a direct effect is lacking.

Between two cultures

The Culture and Identity Schedule turned up trumps. The Asian patients were as adherent to their traditional culture as their controls, or in several areas even more so. The African-Caribbean patients showed a completely different pattern. In two areas, the question of which partner in a relationship should make the decisions, and in the use of patois, the patients were more traditional than their controls. But in four other areas they were significantly less traditional than their controls, indicating that they had moved away from their cultural roots. The areas were: preference for ethnic food, preference to live and work with members of your own ethnic group, leisure activities focused on your own ethnic group, and ethnicity of public figures you admire. In the last area, for example, the patients were more likely than their healthy controls to cite white celebrities as people they admired. It is highly unlikely that they were accepted by the white community whose company they sought and whose values they were beginning to adopt, so that we can assume that they were in the uncomfortable position of having lost some of the support from members of their community but with nothing to replace it. The different pattern from the Asian patients argues that this is not a result of developing schizophrenia, but a possible contributor to the high rate among UK African-Caribbeans. This is a unique finding as no previous study has used a measure of cultural identity in relation to schizophrenia. The finding will have to be replicated in another study before much weight is placed on it, but it is an exciting prospect to have identified a candidate social factor in the causation of schizophrenia.

Separation from parents

One unexpected finding emerged from our analysis. The African-Caribbean patients had more often experienced four or more years of separation from their mother and father in childhood than their controls or than either of the other two groups of patients. This pattern suggests that separation from parents in childhood is specifically linked with the high rate of schizophrenia in the UK African-Caribbean population. But how could it operate to increase the risk of schizophrenia? There are many possible reasons for children being separated from one or both parents, including the development of schizophrenia in a parent and their subsequent admission to hospital. We were able to rule this out as a factor operating in the lives of the patients in our study. We did not enquire into other circumstances leading to separation, but it was quite common for African-Caribbean parents migrating to take up jobs in the UK to leave their children behind in the care of female relatives. After some years, when they felt financially secure and had established a permanent residence, they would send for the children. By this time there were

often other siblings who had been born in the UK. Thus the
children migrating belatedly would have to adapt to parents
they might not have seen for many years and to a substantially
new family. How they had fared in the meantime was also
dependent on the quality of the substitute parenting they
received. These major disruptions in family life and relationships could well have led to problems in forming attach-
ments in adult life. In the previous chapter I quoted Edward
Hare's research in Bristol which showed that the distribution
of schizophrenia in the city was linked with the concentration
of single-person households. It is possible to incorporate these
two observations into a theory that childhood problems in
forming relationships lead to social isolation as an adult
which in turn increases the susceptibility to schizophrenia.

Leroy was born in Jamaica to parents who emigrated to England in
search of jobs when he was three years old. They left him in the
care of one of his mother's sisters who had no children of her own.
She was a strict disciplinarian who discouraged him from playing
with other local children, whom she viewed as too rough. Leroy's
parents established themselves successfully in the Brixton area of
London, his mother working in a local hospital as a nursing assistant
while his father became a train driver. They had three more children
and arranged for Leroy to come to England when he was twelve. He
had great difficulty in making relationships with his brothers and
sister, and became increasingly rebellious. He did not settle into
schooling and regularly truanted on his own. He failed to make
friends with any of his classmates and left school at age fifteen with
no qualifications. After a series of stormy arguments with his father
on account of his lack of occupation, he left home to live in a squat
with a group of other youths who were part of a criminal subculture.
During the next few years he was charged for a number of offences,
mostly shoplifting and damage to property. At age eighteen he was
caught by the police breaking into a store and was remanded in
prison awaiting a trial. A few days later he began to behave strangely,
taking off all his clothes and shouting. He was seen by a psychiatrist

to whom Leroy complained that his cell was bugged and that he heard voices calling him a black bastard. The psychiatrist made a diagnosis of schizophrenia and admitted Leroy to a psychiatric unit.

A link between social networks in childhood and the later development of schizophrenia is supported by findings from longitudinal cohort studies. These are far-sighted endeavours in which all the children born in a particular period in one country are followed up at regular intervals for as many decades as possible. This strategy addresses the problem raised in Chapter 3 that the time unit of interest to the researcher is the lifespan of the subject. By engaging successive teams of researchers to follow up a birth cohort, between them they can keep passing on the Olympic torch, and eventually cover the whole lives of the subjects. This strategy has already thrown some surprising light on the origins of schizophrenia. Children who eventually develop schizophrenia as adults differ from those who do not by their level of sociability. Children with three or fewer friends are at much higher risk of later schizophrenia than those with a larger circle of friends. This has been interpreted as showing that the genes for schizophrenia already exert an influence in childhood by reducing sociability. But an alternative reading is that children who are unable to build a social support system for whatever reason are more vulnerable to the stresses that may provoke an attack of schizophrenia. Our findings for the African-Caribbean patients would fit with this interpretation.

Susceptibility of siblings

In 1994 a paper was published by two British researchers, Philip Sugarman, a psychiatrist, and David Craufurd, a geneticist,[63] which was of signal importance for the controversy between the genetic and environmental theories of schizophrenia in African-Caribbean patients. They conducted a family study of schizophrenia in African-Caribbean and white patients in Manchester. What they found was most surprising. Previous family studies had established that the risk of schizophrenia in the parents of people with schizophrenia is about 10 per cent compared with the general population risk of one per cent. They found the same increased risk in the parents of the patients of both ethnic groups, which is what a geneticist would predict. However, when they looked at the siblings of the patients a very different picture emerged. The siblings of the white patients had a risk of around two per cent, but the risk for the siblings of the African-Caribbean patients was very much higher. For those born in the West Indies the risk was four times that for the white siblings, while for African-Caribbean siblings born in the UK the risk was an astonishing twelve times greater. This finding could be explained by a combination of select- ive migration of people from the West Indies predisposed to schizophrenia, and assortative mating. The latter term accounts for a high incidence of a disease by postulating that people with a predisposition to it are attracted to each other, thereby passing on to their children a much higher risk of developing the disease. In this case, the fact that the parents of the white and African-Caribbean patients had a similar risk for schizophrenia argues against both selective migration and assortative mating, so that a pathogenic influence of the environment on second-generation African- Caribbeans is a more plausible explanation.

So challenging was the finding on family susceptibility that it demanded to be checked as soon as possible. The study was repeated in London in 1995 by an African-Caribbean colleague of ours, Gerard Hutchinson, and his associates.[64] They closely replicated Sugarman's and Craufurd's results. The parents of white and African-Caribbean patients with psychosis had a similar risk of developing the same illness. African-Caribbean siblings born in the West Indies had a slightly higher risk than white siblings, but African-Caribbean siblings born in the UK had a risk seven times that of white siblings. These startling results have focused attention on the environment in which African-Caribbeans in the UK live, but the physical environment is as much suspect as the social environment. Theories have been advanced that African-Caribbean women are more susceptible to virus infections than white women and that the spread of infections in crowded cities could lead to infections during pregnancy which might adversely affect the development of the brain. To date no evidence has been found to support this theory, or the suggestion that African-Caribbean women suffer more complications of pregnancy leading to lack of oxygen at birth. One explanation for our finding of a link between separation from parents and the later development of schizophrenia is that the patient was left behind in the Caribbean as a child. This would seem to conflict with the evidence for the deleterious influence of the living environment on African-Caribbeans born and brought up in the UK. However, just as geneticists now accept that several genes probably act together to produce the susceptibility to schizophrenia, there are likely to be multiple sources of environmental stress that influence the development of the illness.

A search for causative factors in the social environment does not negate the importance of an inherited component to schizophrenia, for which I find the evidence convincing. However, it does challenge the prevailing view of schizophrenia as a purely biological entity. The evidence that social factors influence the course of the disease is now generally accepted (see Chapter 3), so that it does not require a major act of faith to extend the concept of schizophrenia to encompass social causation. The strategy of studying schizophrenia in ethnic minority groups has not indicated for certain what it is about city life that increases the risk of schizophrenia. However, it has identified early separation from parents and uncertainty about cultural identity as possible contributors to the origin of schizophrenia. If indeed these experiences turn out to increase vulnerability to the disease, there is something that can be done about them, which could reduce the risk of developing schizophrenia and save some people from a lifetime of illness.

The Future

There can be no doubt that techniques of monitoring the functioning of the living brain will increase rapidly in sophistication in the near future. It is equally certain that there will be major advances in the application of molecular biology to diseases of the mind. The complete map of the human genome is now available. However, I do not believe that it will ever be possible to explain human behaviour in terms of genes, neurotransmitters, or regional changes in activity of the brain. Human behaviour does not occur in a social vacuum. The psychoanalyst, Donald Winnicott, once made the challenging statement that 'there is no such thing as a baby'. He meant, of course, that a baby cannot survive on its own, but needs the nurture and care provided by other people. In this book I have presented many different studies which illustrate our interdependence as social beings with other people. Only a tiny fraction of the population live in total social isolation by choice. Even were we to consider a Robinson Crusoe, shipwrecked on a deserted island, he would carry with him the history of his relationships with all the important people in his life, with whom he would continue to carry on an internal dialogue. A complete knowledge of his genes would tell us nothing about his ongoing interaction with figures from the past who would people the island.

The complexity of the relationships we establish with other

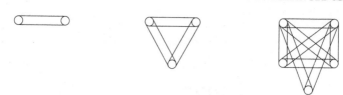

Figure 5 Network of relationships between groups of two, three and five people

people should not be underestimated. While pondering this one day, I realised that there is a simple formula that enables us to calculate the number of relationships generated by the people who are close to us. It is: $n(n-1)$. Two people have $2 \times (2-1) = 2$ relationships, that is, A's relationship with B, and B's relationship with A. If two people have a child together, n becomes 3, and the number of relationships increases to $3 \times (3-1) = 6$ relationships. A couple with three children and their partners have 56 relationships between them. No simple one-to-one correspondence between genes and behaviour could encompass the quantum leap necessary to understand the interactions in even a small social network of people (Figure 5).

The understanding achieved of one level of organisation of the physical world cannot simply be transferred to the next level of complexity. What we have learned about the behaviour of fundamental particles through the development of quantum mechanics does not help us to understand how atoms interact. The characteristic behaviour of atoms gives us no clues as to what to expect from a living cell. From the functional capacity of an individual nerve cell, we could not predict the abilities of the 100 billion neurons that make up the human brain, including the existence of consciousness, the origins of which remain obscure. By the same argument events in the brain – however clearly defined – throw only a dim light on social and emotional interactions between people. Although a group of people has been compared with an organism, the similarities are superficial. Group behaviour can only be understood by studying groups, not by extrapolating from what we know about the behaviour of individuals.

I could have introduced the book with this argument, but you would not then have been in possession of all the evidence presented here that our minds can be unbalanced by disturbances in our social environment, and that the balance can be restored by actively reshaping our relationships with the people who matter to us. I have shown that events in our early life and in recent months determine whether we will become depressed or anxious; that emotional relationships with family members influence the course of a wide range of psychiatric disorders; that skilled work directed at improving these relationships can reduce the risk of relapse for people with depression or schizophrenia; and that the better outcome for schizophrenia in developing countries is largely due to the attitudes of the family towards the patient.

My vision for the future of psychiatry is one that depends not on technical advances in making images of the brain or replacing bad genes with good ones, but on increasing our understanding of relationships between people. It has become starkly clear that industrialisation and urbanisation, those unstoppable forces of modern societies, destroy the extended family and bonds with neighbours which are the essence of traditional ways of life. With the loss of this natural support network, individuals are more vulnerable to psychiatric disorders and it becomes more difficult to restore their mental health. It is useless to issue pleas to retain the extended family, as do some pundits in developing countries. The changes that have already happened in the West are bound to sweep across the rest of the world. The best we can do is to help the reduced nuclear family to cope with psychiatric illness in one of their members by offering skilled professional help as early as possible in its course. This will require a considerable research effort to identify the disturbances in relationships that have contributed to specific psychiatric disorders and the most effective interventions to correct them. The pattern of research needed to do this has already been laid down. Progress will come from achieving the right balance between biological and social research into the complexities of the human mind.

References

1 Leff, J. P., and Wing, J. K. Trial of maintenance therapy in schizophrenia. *British Medical Journal* (1971) **3**, 599–604.
2 Hirsch, S. R., Gaind, R., Rohde, P. D., Stevens, B. C., and Wing, J. K. Out-patient maintenance of chronic schizophrenic patients with long-acting fluphenazine: double-blind placebo trial. *British Medical Journal* (1973) **1**, 633–7.
3 Leff, J. P., Hirsch, S. R., Gaind, R., Rohde, P. D., and Stevens, B. C. Life events and maintenance therapy in schizophrenic relapse. *British Journal of Psychiatry* (1973) **123**, 659–60.
4 Fossey, L., Papiernik, E., and Bydlowski, M. Postpartum blues: a clinical syndrome and predictor of postnatal depression? *Journal of Psychosomatic Obstetrics and Gynaecology* (1997) **18**, 17–21.
5 Kumar, R., and Robson, K. M. A prospective study of emotional disorders in childbearing women. *British Journal of Psychiatry* (1984) **144**, 35–47.
6 Gillis, L. S., Elk, R., Ben-Arie, O., and Teggin, A. The Present State Examination: experiences with Xhosa-speaking patients. *British Journal of Psychiatry* (1982) **141**, 143–7.
7 Orley, J. H., and Wing, J. K. Psychiatric disorders in two African villages. *Archives of General Psychiatry* (1979) **36**, 513–20.
8 Goldberg, D., Cooper, B., Eastwood, M. R., Kedward, H. B., and Shepherd, M. A standardised psychiatric interview for use in community surveys. *British Journal of Social and Preventive Medicine* (1970) **24**, 18–23.
9 Holmes, T. H., and Rahe, R. H. The social readjustment rating scale. *Journal of Psychosomatic Research* (1967) **11**, 213–18.
10 Brown, G. W., and Birley, J. L. T. Crises and life changes and the onset of schizophrenia. *Journal of Health and Social Behaviour* (1968) **9**, 203–14.
11 Brown, G. W., and Harris, T. *The Social Origins of Depression* (Tavistock, London, 1978).

12 Rutter, M. *Maternal Deprivation Reassessed*, 2nd edn. (Penguin, Harmondsworth, 1981).

13 Harrison, J., Barrow, S., Gask, L., and Creed, F. Social determinants of GHQ score by postal survey. *Journal of Public Health Medicine* (1999) **21**, 283–8.

14 Kleinman, A. *Social Origins of Distress and Disease: Depression, Neurasthenia and Pain in Modern China* (Yale University Press, New Haven, 1986).

15 Schwab, M. E. A study of reported hallucinations in a Southeastern County. *Mental Health and Society* (1977) **4**, 344–54.

16 Laing, R. D., and Esterson, A. *Sanity, Madness and the Family*, vol. I: *Families of Schizophrenics* (Tavistock, London, 1964).

17 Hirsch, S. R., and Leff, J. P. *Abnormalities in Parents of Schizophrenics*. Maudsley Monograph 22 (Oxford University Press, London, 1975).

18 Kramer, M. Cross-national study of diagnosis of the mental disorders: origin of the problem. *American Journal of Psychiatry* (1969) **125** (suppl.), 1–11.

19 Cooper, J. E., Kendall, R. E., Gurland, B. J., Sharpe, L., Copeland, J. R. M., and Simon, R. *Psychiatric Diagnosis in New York and London*. Maudsley Monograph 20 (Oxford University Press, London, 1972).

20 Wing, J. K., Cooper, J. E., and Sartorius, N. *The Description and Classification of Psychiatric Symptoms: An Instruction Manual for the PSE and CATEGO System* (Cambridge University Press, London, 1974).

21 Hacking, I. *Rewriting the Soul* (Princeton University Press, Princeton, 1995).

22 Robins, L. N. *Deviant Children Grown Up* (Williams & Wilkins, Baltimore, 1966).

23 Brown, G. W., Carstairs, G. M., and Topping, G. Post hospital adjustment of chronic mental patients. *Lancet* (1958) **ii**, 685–9.

24 Heimann, P. On countertransference. *International Journal of Psychoanalysis* (1950) **31**, 81–4.

25 Brown, G. W., Birley, J. L. T., and Wing, J. K. Influence of family life on the course of schizophrenic disorders: a replication. *British Journal of Psychiatry* (1972) **121**, 241–58.

26 Vaughn, C. E., and Leff, J. P. The influence of family and social factors on the course of psychiatric illness: a comparison of schizophrenic and depressed neurotic patients. *British Journal of Psychiatry* (1976) **129**, 125–37.

27 Hooley, J. M., Orley, J., and Teasdale, J. D. Levels of expressed emotion and relapse in depressed patients. *British Journal of Psychiatry* (1986) **148**, 642–7.

28 Okasha, A., El Akabawi, A. S., Snyder, A. S., Wilson, A. K., Youssef,

I., and El Dawla, A. S. Expressed emotion, perceived criticism, and relapse in depression: a replication in an Egyptian community. *American Journal of Psychiatry* (1994) **151**, 1001–5.

29 Hayhurst, H., Cooper, Z., Paykel, E. S., Vearnals, S., and Ramana, R. Expressed emotion and depression. A longitudinal study. *British Journal of Psychiatry* (1997) **171**, 439–43.

30 Leff, J., Vearnals, S., Brewin, C. R., Wolff, G., Alexander, B., Asen, E., Dayson, D., Jones, E., Chisholm, D., and Everitt, B. The London Depression Intervention Trial. *British Journal of Psychiatry* (2000) **177**, 95–100.

31 Harris, T., Brown, G. W., and Robinson, R. Befriending as an intervention for chronic depression in an inner city population. *British Journal of Psychiatry* (1999) **174**, 219–24.

32 Leff, J. P., and Vaughn, C. The interaction of life events and relatives, expressed emotion in schizophrenia and depressive neurosis. *British Journal of Psychiatry* (1980) **136**, 146–53.

33 McCreadie, R. G. The Nithsdale schizophrenia surveys. An overview. *Social Psychiatry and Psychiatric Epidemiology* (1992) **27**, 40–5.

34 Tarrier, N., Vaughn, C., Lader, M. N., and Leff, J. P. Bodily reactions to people and events in schizophrenics. *Archives of General Psychiatry* (1979) **36**, 311–15.

35 Cooklin, R., Sturgeon, D., and Leff, J. The relationship between auditory hallucinations and spontaneous fluctuations of skin conductance in schizophrenia. *British Journal of Psychiatry* (1983) **142**, 47–52.

36 Goldberg, D., and Huxley, P. *Mental Illness in the Community: The Pathway to Psychiatric Care* (Tavistock, London, 1980).

37 Harvey, Y. K. The Korean *Mudang* as a household therapist. In W. P. Lebra (ed.) *Culture-bound Syndromes, Ethnopsychiatry and Alternate Therapies* (University Press of Hawaii, Honolulu, 1976).

38 Nichter, M. Idioms of distress: alternatives in the expression of psycho-social distress: a case study from South India. *Culture, Medicine and Psychiatry* (1981) **5**, 379–408.

39 Obeyesekere, G. Depression, Buddhism and the work of culture in Sri Lanka. In A. Kleinman and B. Good (eds) *Studies in the Anthropology and Cross-Cultural Psychiatry of Affect and Disorder* (University of California Press, Berkeley, 1985).

40 Hare, E. H. The changing content of psychiatric illness. *Journal of Psychosomatic Research* (1974) **18**, 283–9.

41 Leff, J. P. Psychiatrists' vs. patients' concepts of unpleasant emotions. *British Journal of Psychiatry* (1978) **133**, 306–13.

42 Snaith, R. P., Bridge, J. W. K., and Hamilton, M. The Leeds scale for self-assessment of anxiety and depression. *British Journal of Psychiatry* (1976) **128**, 156–65.

43 Kendler, K. S., Heath, A. C., Martin, N. G., and Evans, L. G. Symptoms of anxiety and symptoms of depression: same genes, different environment? *Archives of General Psychiatry* (1987) **122**, 451–7.

44 Finlay-Jones, R., and Brown, G. W. Types of stressful life events and the onset of anxiety and depressive disorders. *Psychological Medicine* (1981) **11**, 803–15.

45 Taylor, P. J., and Gunn, J. Homicides by people with mental illness: myth and reality. *British Journal of Psychiatry* (1999) **174**, 9–14.

46 Waxler, N. E. Is outcome for schizophrenia better in non-industrial societies? The case of Sri Lanka. *Journal of Nervous and Mental Diseases* (1979) **167**, 144–58.

47 Murphy, H. B. M., and Raman, A. C. The chronicity of schizophrenia in indigenous tropical peoples. *British Journal of Psychiatry* (1971) **118**, 489–97.

48 Karno, M., Jenkins, J. H., De La Selva, A., Santana, F., Telles, C., Lopez, S., and Mintz, J. Expressed emotion and schizophrenic outcome among Mexican-American families. *Journal of Nervous and Mental Diseases* (1987) **175**, 143–51.

49 Faris, R. E. L., and Dunham, H. W. *Mental Disorders in Urban Areas* (Chicago University Press, Chicago, 1939).

50 Hare, E. H. Mental illness and social conditions in Bristol. *Journal of Mental Science* (1956) **102**, 349.

51 Goldberg, E. M., and Morrison, S. L. Schizophrenia and social class. *British Journal of Psychiatry* (1963) **109**, 785–802.

52 Dunham, H. W. *Community and Schizophrenia: An Epidemiological Analysis* (Wayne State University Press, Detroit, 1965).

53 Dauncey, K., Giggs, J., Baker, K., and Harrison, G. Schizophrenia in Nottingham: lifelong residential mobility of a cohort. *British Journal of Psychiatry* (1993) **163**, 613–19.

54 Lewis, G., David, A., Andreasson, S., and Allebek, P. Schizophrenia and city life. *Lancet* (1992) **340**, 137–40.

55 Marcelis, M., Navarro-Mateu, F., Murray, R., Selten, J. P., and van Os, J. Urbanization and psychosis: a study of 1942–1978 birth cohorts in The Netherlands. *Psychological Medicine* (1998) **28**, 871–9.

56 Littlewood, R., and Lipsedge, M. *Aliens and Alienists* (Penguin Books, Harmondsworth, 1982).

57 Hickling, F. W., McKenzie, K., Mullen, R., and Murray, R. A Jamaican psychiatrist evaluates diagnoses at a London psychiatric hospital. *British Journal of Psychiatry* (1999) **175**, 283–5.

58 Bhugra, D., Hilwig, M., Hossein, B., Marceau, H., Neehall, J., Leff, J., Mallett, R., and Der, G. First contact incidence rates in Trinidad and one year follow-up. *British Journal of Psychiatry* (1996) **169**, 587–92.

59 Mahy, G. E., Mallett, R., Leff, J., and Bhugra, D. First contact incidence rate of schizophrenia on Barbados. *British Journal of Psychiatry* (1999) **175**, 28–33.

60 Hickling, F. W., and Rodgers-Johnson, P. The incidence of first contact schizophrenia in Jamaica. *British Journal of Psychiatry* (1995) **167**, 193–6.

61 Bhugra, D., Leff, J., Mallett, R., Der, G., Corridan, B., and Rudge, S. Incidence and outcome of schizophrenia in Whites, African-Caribbeans and Asians in London. *Psychological Medicine* (1997) **27**, 791–8.

62 Selten, J. P., and Sjiben, A. E. S. First admission rates for schizophrenia in immigrants to the Netherlands. *Social Psychiatry and Psychiatric Epidemiology* (1994) **29**, 71–7.

63 Sugarman, P. A., and Craufurd, D. Schizophrenia and the Afro-Caribbean community. *British Journal of Psychiatry* (1994) **164**, 474–80.

64 Hutchinson, G., Takei, N., Fahy, T., Bhugra, D., Gilvarry, C., Moran, P., Mallett, R., Sham, P., Leff, J., and Murray, R. Morbid risk of schizophrenia in first degree relatives of White and African-Caribbean patients with psychosis. *British Journal of Psychiatry* (1996) **169**, 776–80.

Further Reading

Leff, J. *Psychiatry Around the Globe* (Gaskell, London, 1988).

Leff, J., and Vaughn, C. *Expressed Emotion in Families: Its Significance for Mental Illness* (Guilford, New York, 1985).

Parker, I. Qualitative research. In P. Banister, E. Burman, I. Parker, M. Taylor, and C. Tindall (eds) *Qualitative Methods in Psychology: A Research Guide* (Open University Press, Buckingham, 1994, pp. 1–16).

Rose, S. *Lifelines* (Allen Lane, London, 1997).

Warner, R. *Recovery from Schizophrenia: Psychiatry and Political Economy*, 2nd edn. (Routledge, London, 1994).

World Health Organisation. *The International Pilot Study of Schizophrenia*, vol. 1 (WHO, Geneva, 1973).

Index